# BODY AESTHETICS

## Forget The Limits & Get The Body You Want

## Vlad Galbavy

Published In Association With Juggro Ltd

DISCLAIMER: The material in this book is for informational purposes only. This publication contains opinions and ideas of its author and is intended to provide helpful and informative material on the subjects addressed in this publication. It is sold with the understanding that the author and publishers are not engaged in rendering medical, health, or any other kind of personal professional services in the book. The reader should consult their medical/health professional before adopting any of the suggestions in this book.

The author and publisher of this book specifically disclaims any responsibility for any liability, loss or risk, personal or otherwise, which is incurred as a consequence, directly or indirectly, of the use and application of the information contained in this book.

ISBN-13: 978-80-971564-5-9

To Jojo, Jano and Miky for showing me the world of
natural bodybuilding.

"Even though we are many miles apart, we are absolutely on the same page when it comes to the human body. This book is for both the average person looking to get started in physical fitness and for the elite athlete. Enjoy!"

*Stacie Venagro,*
*2013 World Miss Fitness America PRO,*
*Owner of Stacie Venagro Fitness*

"Effective strategies for both fat loss and muscle building regardless of your current physique."

*Matus Valent,*
*Model America 2006 World Championships,*
*Fitness Cover Model*

"An easy read for anyone determined to forget the limits and get the body they want."

*Denisa Lipovska,*
*2013 IFBB European Bikini Fitness Vice Champion,*
*Personal Fitness Trainer*

"A great insight for anyone looking to get into shape, beautifully detailed. A must read for the current generation of keen gym goers!"

*Aaron J Gough,*
*Personal Trainer,*
*Fitness Coach*

# TABLE OF CONTENTS

## Part 1 – Getting Ready

### I. Body Transformation (p.5)



### II. The Inner Game (p.11)



### III. Goal Setting And Planning (p.23)



## Part 2 – The Basics

### IV. Your Body And Training (p.32)

suitable workout frequency / How to plan your workout / What's the best workout length / What's the optimal number of sets / Why to choose a rep range / How to choose appropriate weights / What are heavy weights / Why to work until failure / What are the best rest intervals / What's the optimal movement speed / How to control the movement / How to use the machines / Why you need to tweak something every now and then / How to include your cardio

### IX. Nutrition For Muscle Development (p.82)

What's the role of protein / What are the energy requirements / Why is food quality important / What are a cheat meal and cheat day good for / What's the best meal frequency / How to time your meals / How to boost your appetite / How to prepare your meals / Why you shouldn't use recipes / Why to keep your new eating habits / How can supplements help you

### Part 4 – Fat Loss

### X. Fat Loss Philosophy (p.91)

What's the cause of storing fat / Why is it about carbohydrate overconsumption / What are the roles of insulin and glucagon / How does calorie restriction affect you / What are the two types of fat / What's the difference between fat loss and weight loss / How to measure your body fat / What's the healthy and sustainable body fat percentage limit / Why more muscle means less fat / What's the use of the Transformation Rocket

### XI. Fat Loss Workout Structure (p.100)

Is fullbody training or training split better / Why to use compound movements / Why to use heavy weights / How to choose your rest interval / What's the best rep range / How your body adapts to stress / What's the most appropriate cardio intensity / How to determine the ratio of weightlifting and cardio / When to do your cardio / How to have fun with cardio / Why you need a day off / What's the role of recovery and rest

# Acknowledgements

I would like to thank my Dad for his enormous support and help on this book but, above all, for his belief in me because it has made such a big difference in my life.

I wish to thank my family and friends for their support, encouragement as well as understanding that I chose to spent my free time working on this book so I could share my insights with other people.

I would like to express my gratitude to all people that participated in making of this book:
especially to my editor, Sarah Kean-Price, who's done a fantastic job in perfecting my original manuscript; to Andre Joseph Martin for designing this eye-catching book cover that I hope you all like and for drawing the illustrations; to my beloved aunt Ali for being the first person to give feedback on the manuscript; to my sister Pavlinka who was the first person to support me when I said I would write this book, and to my close friend Ondrej Dobsinsky, who was the first person to apply it's information and get exceptional results from it too!

Finally, I would like to thank Lukas Gonda, Rudolf Simo, Peter Lackovic and Ivan Rohacek for their insights and opinions on fitness and bodybuilding and for helping me to succeed with my own fitness quests.

**Introduction**

Your physique, your choice. It's true for every one of us.

To get the results you want, you need to know how to approach them. This information is precisely what differentiates people with great physiques from everyone else. If you learn the basic principles of working with your body, you can change your physique at whim. The only prerequisites are the right attitude, determination and persistence.

My name is Vlad Galbavy and I'm a London-based, CYQ Level 3 qualified personal trainer and inventor of the successful board game, JUGGRO PT, which both simulates the process of body transformation and allows people to quickly learn about how to make physical changes.

I've devoted a couple of years to fitness and bodybuilding, going from functional training to muscle building and fat loss. I learnt all kinds of things about both and that led me to focusing on just what the difference is between people that achieve their fitness goals and the people that don't.

I've tried lot of things, made lot of mistakes and interviewed lots of people but, in doing so, I've also learned how to achieve amazing results in the shortest time possible by using the most effective training methods. Fitness and bodybuilding simply became my passion and you're reaping the benefits!

I've written this book to share my knowledge and help you get the results you're after. My book is written for everyone that wants to change the appearance of their body;  no matter where you are or how you look. If you've never been to the gym, you'll get the most out of it but it will be equally interesting for people who have been successfully working out for some time.

As you read, you'll get a new view of life and exercise: you will discover how your subconscious affects your success and how you can set up your mindset so you become unstoppable during this challenge; you will learn how your body works and how you can work with it; you will also learn the role of your diet in the whole process and, of course, how to use your diet to achieve results you've only dreamt about.

After reading this book, you should have enough knowledge and drive to embark on the journey of body transformation to get an attractive physique, healthy body, and solid confidence, knowing that, if you really want to achieve something, you can really do it.


Good Luck!

Vlad Galbavy
vlad@juggro.com

www.juggro.com

# Part 1
# Getting Ready

# I. Body Transformation

Imagine you could design your body yourself. Would it look exactly as it looks right now? Lots of people wouldn't say that but there are also those who are more than satisfied with their physique. And that doesn't happen by chance. However you look right now, your body became that way for a reason. Your physique is a reflection of your eating and exercise habits and changing these habits will change the appearance of your body. It's a straight-forward process. All you need to do is to identify your body's particular needs and then use them to make the changes you want. The laws of cause and reaction are always at work. Someone who doesn't get enough physical activity during the day and consumes more food than needed will simply become obese. The obesity is a result of their habits. The same thing applies to thin people. Someone who eats relatively small amounts of food and doesn't pay attention to the quality of the nutrients they consume will simply always be thin. Eating and exercise habits fundamentally influence the appearance of your physique. If you've been worried about yours, then know that you can change it. All you need to do is stop doing what's been causing it to look that way. Change your habits and change them intelligently. Your body will develop its new shape and you'll start to approach the goal you've always wanted to achieve. All it takes is a little bit of determination and a little bit of patience. Both will make all the difference in your quest for a new physique.

## DESIRE

Before you make the first step, you'll need just one more thing to get started and that's the desire to achieve. Desire is at the beginning of every success so, to start your journey, you need to know what you want. Do you want a nice body? The majority of the people do. What do you want to feel when you look at your body? Do you remember how you felt the last time you saw a picture of someone who had successfully transformed their body? Did you talk about this with the people around you? Did you experience feelings of excitement and rushing energy? Those kinds of feelings show where your passion is and you'll feel more of them as you get closer to your goal. The stronger your desire, the bigger the chance you have of succeeding. If your desire is strong enough, you can do whatever you put your mind to. When you really desire something, you'll go after it and you won't stop until you get there. It's at the beginning of every success. It's the thing that won't let you sit on the sofa and watch the television. It's that sense of power that drags you to your goal and won't be silenced until you achieve it. Find the reason for changing your physique and you'll see just how fast things can move when they start with desire.

## FIND YOUR REASON AND LET IT DRIVE YOU FORWARD

Your reason is more important than your approach even. If you know why you want to do something and why it's important, you'll always find a way to do it. There just has to be a strong reason that comes from within. You can be presented with a whole list of reasons as to why it's good to have a healthy, fully-functioning and good-looking body but none of these will necessarily make you take any action. You can rationally understand every single one but this still might not be enough to spark the desire in you. Therefore, your own, personal reason must come from the depths of your soul and, for it to stick, you must experience emotion when it crosses your mind. Knowing your reason will keep you on your journey when you experience obstacles.

People who embark on body transformation often forget why they started in the first place after they've been doing it for a while. Then, when difficulties arrive, they don't see why they should carry on. Your reason gives you a very easy way to avoid this situation. If you ever find yourself flagging and not knowing why you should go on, you have the reason you sought out right at the beginning: the one you identified, developed and focused on, that tells you why you started this journey. Remembering this may well be the only thing you have to do in order to reach your goal. So, ask yourself this question and don't stop asking until you get a meaningful, memorable answer: Why do you want to transform your body?

## PUSH YOUR LIMITS

As we all know, everyone is different and this holds just as true when you start your body transformation. But, there is one thing that we all have in common. We need that feeling of making progress to reinforce our behaviour. That's why you should always try to push your current limits forward. If you intend to lose some fat, you'll be guided by a number on a scale, by your belt girth or your body fat percentage. If you want to build some muscle, you'll be guided by the size of your muscles or the weight that you lift. Any of these limits can be the way to push yourself forward. For instance, one way of pushing your limits would be to do one additional repetition in the gym. Another would be to strive for one extra or one less inch in the right place. Body transformation can give you the opportunity to experience that feeling of overcoming yourself, of allowing yourself to achieve goals that weren't within your reach before. You'll get to know yourself better than you ever have and you will learn that, actually, there are no limits in life when you put your mind to it. With this knowledge, you get to ask yourself the all-important question: "If I'm able to change the appearance of my body, what else can I achieve?" Overcoming each limit on your journey will prove to you that you are capable of achieving goals; no matter how daring, improbable or difficult they first seemed.

## ILLUSION OF LIMITATION

If you haven't had much chance to challenge your limits, you're probably one of the many people that think there are some things they never achieve. Personal limitations that will never allow them to come out of their shadow. These people reject their chances for success before they've even tried. Instead of looking for ways to do something, they look for reasons to prove that it can't be done. Don't let yourself become one of those people. The only limitations that exist are those that you create in your mind. We can always find a way around a challenge, no matter how impossible it seems. It's part of what makes us human. If you really want something, you can and will do it, regardless of what it is. If you want to get stronger and build some muscle, then look for a way to do it and ignore the limitations your mind throws up before you. If you apply yourself and just keep pushing yourself forward, one step at a time, you'll soon get to what you wanted. If you truly want to lose fat, the same applies. Set up a goal and go after it diligently, refusing to allow your limits to hamper you. Even if your goal seems unachievable right now, this doesn't mean that it can't be achieved. Many people get intimidated by their goals, not realising that this sense of intimidation is the very thing that limits them most. Remember that the achievement of a big goal is nothing but the result of achieving smaller consecutive steps and these are things that can be achieved by anyone.

## INSIGHT INTO THE FUTURE

Start developing yourself now. Think about how your time can work for you. It can be your friend or your foe. It all depends on how you use it. Decide to transform your body now and time will become your friend. If your brain insists you can't do something right now, don't listen to it and don't postpone that goal. Most likely, you won't get a chance to get back to it later. What will happen instead is that, one day after nothing has changed, you'll say, "If I only started back then, I'd look completely different now. I'd feel completely different and I wouldn't have to still deal with this problem". Imagine this scenario and try to immerse yourself in it. Imagine the place you'd be in, imagine the people surrounding you and the conversation that led to you talking about it. Observe the feelings that come with the fact that you stayed inactive instead of striving for change: the feelings of hopelessness, impotence and regret. It definitely doesn't feel good. Remember that action is imperative. Do not postpone your body transformation under any circumstances because, at the end of the day, you'll regret it. Push yourself to challenge one more limit or goal. Don't wait until you have to say, "If I could only get the time back and have one more chance to make a decision!" This is your chance. Grab it with both hands and start your transformation now.

## DECISION

Everything comes down to the choice between two options. The first option is that you continue to merely dream about your amazing body and fail to achieve it. Every New Year, you'll resolve to work on your physique but you'll never get properly started. Then, when summer comes and you want to look good in your swimwear, you'll start going to the gym again, lose a few pounds, stop, regain them and nothing will ever really change. This will go on and on until you become totally complacent about the situation and proclaim that you don't even care about how your body looks. You'll lower your expectations and be absolutely fine with failure, embracing your inability to push your limits. There's another option. Learn how to build your body and start working on yourself. Start right now and the first results will come sooner than you expect. Those first changes, will then give you the appetite to go on. Your physique will visibly change and your progress will be noticed by others as well. The result of your hard work will be a strong and healthy-looking body. You have a choice to make and the decision can only ever be yours. Only you can be responsible for your choices; no one else is or ever can be. Pluck up the courage and seize the new challenge that's been waiting for you.

## YOU CAN DO IT, JUST AS OTHERS HAVE

If you still have doubts about your ability to make the change, then remember you're not the only one with this feeling of uncertainty. It's been experienced by hundreds of thousands of people right across the world. Everyone has the same questions: Do I really want to go through with this? Will it work? Isn't it just a waste of time? Can I really manage it? These questions are absolutely normal and everyone has them, over and over again. When you talk to people that have successfully transformed their body, lots of them will tell you it was a leap in the dark but that, ultimately, they were successful. They got used to their new diet, learned what to do in the gym, worked hard and, one day, looked into the mirror and saw a new person. They had to face some obstacles just like anyone else but they overcame them and carried on. They had to force themselves to go to the gym when they were overwhelmed by other responsibilities or when they just didn't want to. Ultimately, they still got what they aimed for and so will you. If you want to read about similar experiences of overcoming fear and reluctance, then do some research online for other people's stories about their body transformations. You'll be amazed at how many situations you'll find that relate to how you're feeling right now. Take these stories and make the people involved your role models. Perhaps one day, you'll be the same for someone who finds your story during their own internet search!

## WHAT MATTERS TO YOU, NOT EVERYONE ELSE

As you start on your journey, not everyone will try to inspire and support you. There will always be naysayers so you need to be careful when talking to them. When you publicly announce that you intend to transform your body, you'll get all kinds of feedback. Within the group of people you tell, there'll always be those that fear change and try to discourage you. It might be a friend who decided to do something with her body two years ago but she was weak-willed and quit after two weeks, announcing it was impossible. Or a cousin who wanted to gain some muscle in the past but didn't eat adequately, making it an unrealistic goal for him. There will always be people like this and you should be prepared for that. This doesn't mean that you should keep your goal to yourself. Quite the opposite! Share your vision with everyone around you. Some might be able to help you and some will want to join you. But never let anyone decide whether you can transform your body or not. It's your body and no-one else's. Expect the negative feedback and prepare for it but always stay strong. Don't let others drain your willpower and change your decisions. When faced with these negative people, just smile, thank them for their advice and hold on to your vision. They probably don't know anything about exercise, will-power or making this kind of commitment anyway. If you learn how to handle negative comments early on, the path to your new body will be much easier.

## II. The Inner Game

Your mind is one of the most complicated things in this world and it is absolutely critical that you understand it, control it and utilise its full potential. Without preparation, it can become your biggest obstacle. When times are difficult, it will convince you that you are too uncomfortable and discourage you from working on your change, making it likely that you'll give up. The important thing to realize is that your body transformation is not going to be easy. You need to understand why situations like this occur and how you can prepare for them. This chapter has the information to understanding both. There are also tools to help you work with your mind and you'll discover why learning is the best protection against failure. Finally, we'll talk about the Transformation Rocket. This tool will be of tremendous help to you throughout your body transformation.

## SOCIAL PRE-CONDITIONING

Like everyone else, you were born into a society that influences you. Your parents, your neighbours, your friends and even the ice cream vendor! All of them shape and add to the environment that you live in. "This is common sense!", you might say, but our environment has a tendency to shape our personality and it's important that you think about just what it's taught you. In your brain, there are a type of cell called mirror neurons. These mirror neurons cause you to copy behaviours in your environment. For example, have you ever been to a place where a different dialect is used and caught yourself mimicking it? This is exactly the kind of thing that mirror neurons are responsible for. They make you copy the patterns in your environment and are also responsible for your behaviour, your belief systems and your habits. The important thing, however, is that your mind is constantly able to be reprogrammed; the mirror neurons mean that it will change when you expose yourself to something new.  The reason I'm stressing this is that you will experience lots of new things during your body transformation. These things are unlikely to be part of your typical information environment so your mind will start to scream things like: "Why are you doing this? Exercising is hard. Who do you think you are? You don't do things like this! Just sit down and watch a movie!". It wants to stick to what it's used to and this will present additional challenges. The effect of your previous pre-conditioning and the belief systems it lead to makes new starts especially tricky.

## BELIEF SYSTEMS

If you want to reprogramme your brain, you first need to change your belief systems. This is where it all starts. The information you've collected during your lifetime builds the base for your beliefs. Your beliefs are the base of your belief systems and your belief systems affect your decisions. Let's use an example to illustrate this process: John wants to build a muscular body but someone tells him it can't be done naturally so John starts to believe this. He decides that working out is a waste of time and won't start at all because he's been fed information that tells him it's impossible. The fact that he can't build a muscular body naturally is not true but that doesn't matter. John forms the belief that it can't be done, this becomes an established belief system and so he makes his decision based on what he believes rather than the truth. Our belief systems have a serious influence on our behaviour. If you keep to the same belief systems, you'll make the same decisions and therefore get the same results. It works the same with your physique. If you don't change your approach, you will look the same or perhaps even worse.  If you truly want to change the appearance of your physique, you need to go deeper and change some of your beliefs. To do this, you need to change your belief systems and, for that, you need some new information.  The more information you have, the better it's going to be for you.


## YOU AGAINST YOU

Making your start is one of the hardest battles in your journey and the trouble doesn't stop there. Your body transformation will take time and there's a particular obstacle that'll make you feel uncomfortable for part of it. Say hello to your biggest obstacle to success which is you! Consider this: You're getting ready for the gym and, all of a sudden, you remember you have to send a letter you were supposed to send last week. Instead of going to the gym, you go to the post office and you're forced to skip your workout. Why did this happen? Because your time management is weak. Find a way to improve it. Get a book about time management. Get a diary, get an app, get a note pad or whatever's best for you. If you organize your time better, you can't give your brain the excuse to avoid exercise. Learn how to leverage your mind and everything will become easier.


## NO EXCUSES

If you're not in control of your mind, it will start to control you. You'll start making excuses. The most frequent excuse these days is a lack of time and that's just the beginning. My stomach is full. I'm exhausted. It's too hot. It's too cold. It's raining. I don't feel like it. My car is broken. I didn't sleep well. I don't like sweating. I don't know where my keys are. I can't find my socks... The list never ends. It is important to realise that excuses will get you nowhere and that, by giving in to them, they cause a big problem. Do something once and the chances are that you'll do it again. And from there on, the bad habit is formed even though you won't notice it. This habit will stay with you later on, sneaking in and draining your motivation. So, forget about excuses and work hard on yourself. If you really want something, you'll do whatever it takes. You decided you wanted a new body so commit to that. If you make excuses, the only person that suffers the consequences are you. Results don't come easily. You need to work hard to get them. If you're making excuses and not working hard, you won't get your results. Guaranteed. You'll stay where you are and nothing will change. If you really want to transform your body, there's nothing big enough to stop you from doing it.


## BE CAREFUL ABOUT THE WORDS YOU USE

Excuses bring another danger. The way you speak becomes a self-fulfilling prophecy and you must be careful. If you keep telling yourself that you have no time, you'll find that you really don't have time to exercise. But if instead you ask yourself how to find the time needed, you'll start looking for ways how to make it and, suddenly, you'll have it. Your words have power and the ones you choose to use reveal the way you perceive your reality too. A fat person will say to themselves: "I'll never lose weight. I'll always stay fat. I think it's just inevitable, I must be one of those people that can't lose weight." A skinny person will say: "No matter what I do, I just can't put on any weight. I'm eating normally and working out all day long and I still haven't developed any muscles so what's the point?" You don't pick your words randomly. Your words reflect your thoughts and what you think about each day make you who you are. So, if you're thinking about your body, think positively. If you don't like your body now, think about how it will look like in the future. If you're talking about your physique, don't complain about your current state. Instead, tell people about your plan to transform your body. If you're talking about your body negatively, just stop. Notice what you say and start talking about your body positively.

## KNOWLEDGE IS THE BEST PROTECTION

Next, focus on acquiring new knowledge. It affects your belief systems and is the best protection against making the bad decisions that come from how you used to think about your body. A good understanding of how your body works gives you a firm ground for your choices. It also protects you from the various "experts" in your gym. When someone approaches you, telling you should start taking L-Arginin, how will you react? Your reaction will be determined by the level of your awareness and knowledge about exercising, nutrition and supplements. It will help you to recognize good advice from bad. Not only that, but it's fundamental to your transformation. If you understand the cause of bodily changes, you can control them. You need to know as much as possible on the subject of body transformation. It will protect you from mistakes that others make and it will help you maximise your own results as well.

## KEEP ASKING

Every time you discover something you're unfamiliar with, do some research. Approach it like a child. Children are always curious and if they don't understand, they question it. If they don't understand the explanation, they ask again. Do the same thing. Be curious and always keep asking. What training is the best for muscle development? What supplements are most effective after your workout? What do you need to avoid in a gym? What can you expect during the first week of your journey?  Ask anything that interests you. Ask your personal trainer, read books and search the internet. The more information you have, the more effectively you can train. If you have enough information, you'll know how to maximize your results in the shortest time possible. If you have the answers you need, you can relax, knowing that you're doing the right thing. However, make sure that the information you have is high-quality and actually correct. It's not enough to ask once and accept the first answer. The answer may be correct; it may not be. What I recommend is to take an eclectic approach to learning. Consult multiple sources, read around and ask others on the same journey. Compare the answers, think about what's realistic and about others' motivations for believing certain ideas and then decide which answer is the most sound.

## QUALITY OF INFORMATION

Lot of information lacks quality. So how do you know high quality information when you see it? The first thing to do is to examine the source of the information and the second is to always double check the most important information. If you follow nonsense for too long, you won't end up where you want to be and your body won't look as you hoped. Every time that someone gives you advice about your workout, nutrition or supplementation, think about it. Who is it that's giving me this advice? Are they walking the walk or just talking the talk? What results are they getting from it? What do they stand to gain if I follow this advice? Make sure they practice what they preach and before you follow anything: research, check and double-check. If you're still not sure, it's time to ask a professional.


## A PERSONAL TRAINER AND HIS ROLE

Knowledge can be acquired simply by investing time and research and, generally, you'll be able to find what you need relatively quickly. However, it does take time to put the information into practice and to get useful experience. If you want to speed up this process, consider hiring a personal trainer. However, be careful when you're choosing one. You need a personal trainer that's experienced what you're about to experience. Someone that's been in your situation and tested their knowledge of fitness and bodybuilding on their own body. Make sure that they've discovered what does and doesn't work. That they're someone who's travelled the path you want to take and can use that experience to help you achieve the same.  When you've found the right trainer, make sure you can trust them, work closely with them and follow their advice. A good personal trainer will pass on their experiences and will watch and guide you on your way. Their job is also to explain how things work. This is important because if you understand why you need to do something in a certain way rather than another, you will be more invested in doing things correctly. You need to understand why you're doing a certain number of repetitions, why your sleep is so important, why is your post-workout meal important and a whole number of other things. The trainer's job is to explain as much of fitness and bodybuilding as they can. One day you'll find yourself at a level where you won't need them any more and you'll be able to rely on yourself. This is where the trainer's advice, knowledge and experience comes into its own. You'll be working with their methods to continue your journey as an individual. Make sure the trainer you choose can be trusted to have the right information and to explain things well because, further down the road, you'll be working with what they told you.

## SPECIFIC THINKING

Apart from your knowledge and awareness, there's another fundamental part to your transformation; your discipline and morale. There are certain moments when your knowledge can't help you at all. Not yours, not your trainer's, nor anyone else's. You know that you should get ready for your workout and you know what to do in the gym but you just don't feel like working out. You're tired or you're fed-up or you're bored of it all...something's just wrong. Remember, that this is happening only in your head and you simply have to deal with it. Let's consider a time when this happens. Your workout is approaching and you are still tired from your previous day. The worst question you can ask yourself now is: "Do I feel like working out today? Am I in the mood?". Your mind will immediately start looking for everything related to your workout and is uncomfortable about it. You'll imagine struggling and sweating whilst your neighbour barbecues in the garden and so, of course, your answer will be no. The first strategy against procrastination and laziness is to not think about uncomfortable feelings. If you need to work out to achieve your bodily changes then the chances are that you will experience situations like this. On the other hand, if you like exercising and are looking forward to every workout, it shouldn't be much of a problem, even though you'll still find yourself thinking similar things. The second strategy is to instead think about the reward that exercising offers you. Specifically focus on something that brings you pleasure. Think about how good you feel after your workout when you're pumped full of endorphins and feel like you could run for miles. That feeling when you're satisfied with yourself. That moment when you manage to stretch your limits. It could be lifting heavier weights, completing an additional round in your local park, a decrease in your body fat percentage or simply a look in the mirror. Think hard about that pleasurable experience and your motivation will soar. If for some reason that's not the case for you, use the third strategy: think about the pain that follows when you don't work out. Think about the results that laziness brings. That painful feeling in the evening when you're angry with yourself for giving in to your sloth. That sense of disappointment as your body feels flabbier, rather than toned.  Whatever you feel when you fail to stick with your goals, take that as your motivation.

## MAKE THE FIRST STEP

There is one more excellent strategy that can help you and it's pretty simple: just make the first step. This works in any arena of your life and I strongly suggest trying it. If you don't feel like going to gym, fine. Instead, just stand up and start packing your stuff. It's a simple task. It won't take you much time and it's useful because, hey, whenever you do want to go, it'll be packed and ready, right? Once you've done that, you can feel pleased with yourself because you did what you said you'd do. Hold on to that feeling of positivity. Now that you've completed that task, it would be rather a shame if you didn't go to the gym, wouldn't it?  Pick up your bag, go to the door and get out of your house. If you walk for a couple of streets and find that you seriously don't want to work out today, you can still turn around and go back home. After all, it's your choice. You're just taking the opportunity to make sure what you're feeling is actually true. What's so good about this method is that you will probably finish your journey, work out and go home again. Basically, we humans are horrible at making changes. If we start to do something, we are most likely to continue doing it because our brains don't want to change gear. So try to leverage this and use it in your fight against procrastination and laziness. You can sit in front of your laptop literally any other time of the day. It won't hurt to take an hour out. Quite the opposite, in fact!

## TRANSFORMATION ROCKET

At the beginning of this chapter, I promised you a description of the Transformation Rocket and here it is. The Transformation Rocket is simply a tool that depicts the process of body transformation. Every body transformation consists of the same requirements. Every person that has gone through, is going through or will go through body transformation needs to meet six basic requirements to be successful in this endeavour. These are decision, discipline, time, training, nutrition and supplementation. Think of these as individual engines that move the rocket forward. If all six engines work properly, the rocket will get to its destination directly without any delays. But, if one or more engines don't work properly, the rocket will diverge from its planned course and will arrive at its destination either late or not at all. If you meet all six requirements for body transformation, you will achieve your results in the time expected. If you neglect one or more requirements, your transformation will take longer or, worse, not happen at all. So, use every one of the six engines the Transformation Rocket needs to control your progress. It will save you hours of wasted work.

## SIX ENGINES

Each engine of the Transformation Rocket symbolizes one of the mentioned requirements. Let's have a look at what these requirements represent.

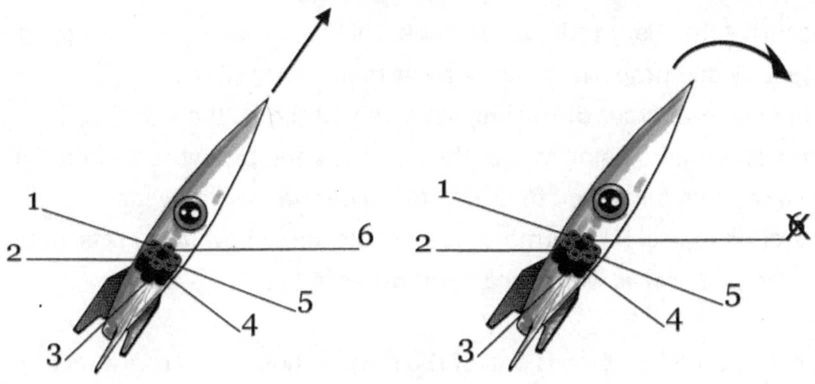



*1. Decision 2. Discipline 3. Time 4. Training 5. Nutrition 6. Supplementation*

1. Decision – Every change begins with a big decision. However, as we discussed, your decision must come from an inner belief that no other option than change is acceptable. You know your body deserves the change but you must be fuelled by an inner power. It is not enough to say you want to transform your body. You need to be 100% committed to this decision you've made.

2. Discipline – Can you constantly work on your goals? It's not enough to train every now and then and to have a chicken salad for dinner every now and then. You need to approach your plan with discipline and stick to it at all times. Daily discipline is an assurance that you will achieve your new physique.

3. Time – Your body transformation requires an investment of time. You must allocate time to training, meal preparation and other things. It just won't work without it. You also need to realise that you won't get quick results. Your body will start to change over the course of several weeks and so you need to be patient to see this happen. Time is a very important part of the Transformation Rocket.

4. Training – Your body change will occur as your body reacts to the incentive that your training provides. This means that you need to train regularly and properly. It's important to understand the specific influence that types of training have on your body, the workout principles you're going to use, the exercises and proper technique for each of them and when to use certain exercises and how many exercises to use. Furthermore, you should know how many sets and reps to perform as well as plenty of other things.

5. Nutrition – Nutrition is one of the most important factors affecting the appearance of your body. Without proper nutrition, you'll get nowhere. You can have discipline, go to the gym, work out and sleep well but if you don't have decent nutrition, changes can't occur.

6. Supplementation – The last but equally important engine is supplementation. Supplements will help you get the maximum results which is why you need to know as much about them as possible. You need to know which supplements can help you and which supplements are worth the money.

## KEEP A BALANCE BETWEEN ALL ENGINES

The last thing to mention is that it's important to keep all your engines balanced once you've embarked on your body transformation journey. The performance of each and every one affects the others. Strive to meet all six requirements, find the balance between them and make sure you don't neglect any of them. If you find a weakness, work on it until it vanishes. If you understand all six engines and master the power of this tool, your body transformation will be easier than you think.

# III. Goal setting and planning

To achieve something, you first need to know what exactly you want and you need to set particular goals. Someone who doesn't set any goals for themselves is easily manipulated. If you want to be successful, you need to keep an eye on your dreams, measure your progress and keep moving forward. Why is this so important? Again, it's related to how your mind works. Your mind focuses on two things: pain and pleasure. It is always looking for a way to avoid the former and maximise the latter. Not only that but it only considers your current situation and is not overly concerned about the future. Therefore, if you don't set up any goals for your mind to focus on, it will only work with impulses within the present. However, if you set up goals, your mind will start focusing on their achievement in the long term and the delayed pleasure this will bring. Immediate pain and pleasure will become a secondary concern instead. Clearly define your goals in a useful fashion and it will be easier for you to keep on course and to constantly move forward.

**BAD GOALS**

Lots of people understand the importance of goal setting but they don't choose the right goals. Theirs are unclear and unmeasurable which is a recipe for failure. Let's have a look at what bad goals look like:
"I want to build some muscle."
"I want to lose some fat."
"I want to have an attractive butt."
"I want to look like a model."
"I want to have a wide back."
All these goals are set up for failure because their progress tracking is based on opinion. One day it'll seem like you're a million years from your goal and the next week, you'll feel like you can proclaim your goal

achieved. When talking about personal issues, people tend to see things unclearly. They tend to look at themselves in the best light possible because their ego loves this. Therefore, a goal based on opinion, mood and point of view will get you nowhere. It might work as a reason for your decision but it is very ineffective as a goal. You need to set up goals which will give you a sound base for tracking your progress.

## NEED FOR MEASUREMENT

Regardless of what you're measuring, tracking your progress always requires numbers. Let's have a look at some good indicators. The first is your bodyweight. Your bodyweight will nearly always be different at the beginning and at the end of each month during your body transformation. Sometimes this number will halt, even though you are making progress. When you work out, a certain amount of your fat is replaced by a certain amount of new muscle tissue and even though your bodyweight stays the same, your body composition does change. People get usually confused with this and they start wondering if they're doing everything as they're supposed to. However, remember that your bodyweight is not the only indicator of your progress. It is necessary to measure other important things as well. Measure your body fat percentage and your body part circumferences. These will give you a complete image of your physique and avoid confusion when your weight temporarily stops changing. Similarly, be sure to measure the weight of resistance you use and the time spent on cardio.  These indicators are explained later in the following chapters and you'll see how they are a way of measuring your caloric intake and expenditure. Remember that to be effective, your goals must be measurable and usable at all times.

## GOOD GOALS

So, to stay on your path, determine the attributes you want to measure regularly and then measure them. Don't forget that your goal is to achieve particular numbers because all good goals contain measurable numbers:

"I will lose 2 inches from my waist by the end of May."

"I will be able to do 10 reps in a set of pull ups by Christmas."

"I will lose 3% body fat in a month"

"I will lose 10 pounds by the beginning of July"

Did you notice that I used numbers in every example? You need to do the same. Find out where you are now and where you want to go. You need to know your current bodyweight, your body fat percentage, your waist circumference and your thigh and arm circumferences. Start by measuring everything and make sure to keep measuring yourself all the way through your body transformation. When you have everything measured, set up some goals for yourself. Decide how much you want to weigh, the body fat percentage you want and the desired body part circumferences. However, be careful to choose goals that are realistic. Some people would like to lose 50 pounds in 20 days or increase their chest circumference by 4 inches in a week but that's just not going to happen. Set up realistic goals and realistic numbers that you can start working towards progressively.

## NO RANGE ALLOWANCE

In setting your goals, it's important to be specific. It's not enough to say you are going to lose 10 to 15 pounds in 30 days. Will it be 10lbs or 15lbs? Decide. Your goals must be set up completely clearly. If you think that 15 pounds is too much for now, go for 10 pounds. When you achieve that, you can set a new goal and lose those other 5 pounds as well. So focus on just one number. Your mind is more able to focus on a clear command, rather than vague ideas. If you set up a particular target, it can take you straight to it. This is why you need particular numbers and in this case, those numbers are your bodyweight, body fat percentage and the circumferences of your body parts. If you don't have these numbers yet, now is the time for you to get them.  Find out what they are now and decide what you want to get to. Just remember that those numbers must be specific.

## WRITE IT DOWN

Once you set up your goals and you know exactly what you want, write it down on paper. This step is very important so make sure you don't skip over it. Your goals need to be recorded somewhere clearly and simply. Write them on paper, on your laptop or on your mobile phone because you will probably forget them soon enough. Right now, they're on your mind and your short term memory is working with them but everything will be different in a month. Don't try to act like a hero; just write them down. Once you've written them down, you'll remember that moment clearly and you'll become more committed to go after them until you achieve them and your vision becomes reality.

## ADD A DATE TO YOUR GOALS

The last thing you need to do for perfect goal-setting is to add a specific date of when you want to have achieved your goals. Write it right next to those goals you've just written down. Again, choose a realistic date and don't choose deadlines that are impossible to meet. You'll only get discouraged and you really don't want that. If you want to lose 5lbs of fat for example, give yourself at least 2 weeks depending on your situation. Don't expect to lose it in 3 days. Choose a date that will allow you to move forward but won't put too much pressure on you either. However, don't give yourself excessive time margins either because this is no holiday. Decide on a date that will push you forward and keep you active. If you don't know how to determine one, think about how close you can be to achieving your goals in a week, two weeks or a month. Think about what is realistic for you and you will find the right date you need in no time. If you're lost in these assumptions, I'll give you an example. The optimal speed of losing fat is about 1 pound a week even though it can be more so if you want to lose 10lbs of fat, it might take you about 10 weeks if you do things right. However, leave yourself some space for mistakes and set your deadline for 11 weeks. You never know which obstacles you'll encounter.

## IDENTIFY POSSIBLE OBSTACLES

Now that your goals are down in ink, let's move on to the second part. Identify the obstacles that may come your way during your transformation. Obstacles always arise and your reaction will depend on how prepared you are. If you identify obstacles ahead of time, you can get ready for them. You've probably heard this quote before: Expect the best but prepare for the worst. Don't let yourself get into a situation where you encounter an obstacle and you don't have a plan for it. Make a list of every possible obstacle you could encounter. If you know what obstacles might show up, you can create a detailed plan of how to overcome them. First, focus on your daily activities. How are you going to handle them whilst investing enough time into your body transformation? How will you manage to spend enough time with your family and friends? Will you have enough time for your hobbies? How will you travel to the gym? What will you do if you get stuck at work all day? Furthermore, think about obstacles related directly to your body transformation. How will you ensure your meals are always ready? How often will you increase your workload? What supplements are you going to use? Lastly, think about obstacles that you create for yourself. How will you beat your laziness and procrastination? How will you ensure you don't cut corners? Address these questions now and get ready for them. It'll save your time in the long run.

## CREATE A PLAN

Let's get started now! Take an obstacle and think about what you'll do
to overcome it. For example, it's 3pm and your workout is scheduled
for 6pm. However, your boss comes in and unexpectedly asks you to
stay at work until 7pm. The project you're working on has experienced
some unexpected complications so you agree and decide to stay. You
had planned to go to the gym at 6pm. However, you were expecting
this possible obstacle and you have a plan for a situation like this.
Instead of going to gym at 6pm to work out for an hour, you do a home
workout at 8pm and cut the workout down to 40 minutes. Instead of no
workout, you cover the basic exercises. It's always better to have
a shorter workout than to have no workout at all. A shorter workout
will leave space for other things that were on your agenda that day too.
The important thing is that you weren't surprised by the obstacle and
that you knew how to react because you had a plan. So, have a look at
each and every one of those obstacles you identified and create a plan
on how to overcome them one by one. You need to be prepared.

## CREATE NEW GOALS

Now that your goals are set up and your plan for overcoming obstacles
is designed, I wish you every bit of success and fun on your way to
achieving your goals! Work on yourself diligently and soon you will get
to where you want to be. The next question, however, is where to go
from there. Will you revert to your previous habits, maintain your
current state or will you accelerate your goals? It would be a shame to
return to where you began and you'd certainly regret it. If you find
yourself satisfied with how your new body looks like, maintain it. You
won't need to work as hard as during your body transformation. Once

your goals have been attained, you only need to work out two to three times a week and watch your nutrition. But why not see just how far you can get? Why not work on yourself a bit more? It won't be that difficult now. You're familiar with it now and you have momentum too. Rather than discarding all that hard work when you reach your current goals, set up new ones and keep moving forward. I explained it at the beginning of this chapter, goal setting is very important. Without goals, you're like a leaf that the wind can blow wherever it wants, with no control and no idea of what will happen. Set up some new goals and direct your steps towards their achievements. You will not regret it, I can promise you that!

## MASSIVE AND CONSTANT ACTION

I would like to remind you of one more thing that is very important. Dreaming and planning are not enough for your body transformation. You need to commit to massive and constant action. You need to start acting and then not stop, no matter the circumstances that life throws up. If you already know what to do, start working on yourself. If you don't have enough information to start with your body transformation, keep reading and focusing on acquiring new information. Read about how to design a workout programme, what to eat and how to work out. Watch some videos. Start looking for a personal trainer. If you're not working out because you're reading up on the subject, you're still taking meaningful action. However, be careful not to get stuck in a reading loop. No one ever transformed their body by reading books or watching videos online and, at some point, you have to actually put the theory into practice. Start going to the gym and get used to the gym environment. Get familiar with the exercises that you'll be using during your body transformation. Learn how to perform them correctly. Ask someone to help you if you need it. If you're completely new to the world of fitness and bodybuilding, your learning curve will be very steep and perhaps a little intimidating. However, it won't take too long and you will feel comfortable in the gym. Remember that every step forward counts, even when it's a small one.

## DO SOMETHING EVERY DAY

Always push yourself to learn a little more. When you've finished reading this book, start reading another one or watch some videos online. Have a little workout. Or perhaps today is your day off so no workout? No problem. Search online, find another success story and get inspired. Occupy yourself everyday with something that can get you a little closer to your goal. Keep this connection with your goal. Regularity plays a very important role in this. If you occupy your mind with your transformation every day, you'll maintain a valuable momentum. Each day spent adding to your momentum will see your efforts multiply and you'll get better results. If you're tempted to slacken your tempo, just imagine what would you have to go through to get back to it again. Remember how hard it was to get to this point? So, don't lose contact with your training and enthusiasm for your body transformation. Just keep doing something for your body every day and you will be surprised at the results you can achieve and how swiftly you reach them!

## NEVER GIVE UP

As the chapter closes, I want to tell you that I do appreciate your body transformation comes with a certain level of challenge; perhaps unlike anything you've ever done. But never forget there is an ultimate reward waiting for you at the end of this journey: a healthy, strong and attractive body. Just be aware that those results don't come easily and you need to persevere until the end. An enormous percentage of people fail to persevere and give up at the first major obstacle. This usually happens when they don't see any results. However, you can avoid all this. If your results don't appear, there are only two things that can have caused it. You either haven't invested enough time into your body transformation or you're doing something wrong. Your training might be wrong, your nutrition might be wrong or both of them might be wrong. Don't stop just because of a lack of results. Take that frustration and use its energy to think about the possible mistakes you're making and correct them instead. Accept the fact that you've made a mistake and start again. There's nothing to feel bad about after all, you're just learning a new skill. It's easy to quit but it's difficult to live knowing that you gave up at the first hurdle. So, if you don't manage to achieve your goals in the time you expected, don't take it as failure. The chances are that you were a good 80% of the way to completing your goal anyway. You just need to tweak your method. Rather than focus on 'failure', be proud of the progress you've made. Although you haven't gotten to your goal in the expected time, it's likely just a question of several days' more work. There's no reason to give up. Being tired, not hitting your targets exactly or finding it difficult simply aren't good enough reasons for you to give up and everything you're experiencing is a normal part of change. Just stay on your path and don't give up; after all, you've come so far already.

# IV. Your body and training

The more you know your body, the easier it is for you to get a specific reaction. It is easier for you to lose some fat if you know what's happening in your body and it's easier to build some muscle if you know what your body responds to positively. You simply need to know how your body functions. After all, it's a complex system and lot of things relate to each other. This chapter will tell you about the different things affecting your system: genetics, physical composition, muscle tissue, the way it reacts and how to work with what you've got. Take time to learn the basic principles about how your body functions and how to change its appearance in a way that you want. The basic principles will be beneficial for you whatever your goal and this understanding will give you long-term assurance and confidence when working with your body.

## GENETICS

The very first thing that you need to know about is genetics. You can't influence your genetics but they influence you. If your parents are both around 160cm tall, you're never going to be 200cm.  Everyone knows that genetics affects their height, skin colour, eye colour and other similar things. However, genetics influence your muscles development capability as well. Your muscles can be developed only as far as your genetics allow. Moreover, when you start working out, you'll find that some body parts respond to your training exceptionally well and that some of them are very challenging. This too is caused by genetics but don't let that become your excuse. When you focus your effort towards those body parts a little more and find out what is working for them, you'll easily solve the problem. Another thing influenced by genetics is your growth potential. Everyone has a certain genetic potential for their growth. With natural body-building, you will get to a point when you won't be able to improve any further; this is when you know you've achieved your genetic potential. This potential represents a final barrier to your body transformation because there will be an upper limit to how far you can go. So, genetics really do influence the appearance of your physique. Luckily, it doesn't critically influence the majority of your body transformation. If you strive to build muscle, you will gradually build it and if you strive to lose fat, you will lose it. This doesn't depend on genetics but on your training, nutrition and supplementation.

## BODY COMPOSITION

When you work on your body transformation, you're working with your body composition which is a ratio of body fat, bones and muscle. This is best understood by an example. Take two people of the same height and same weight standing next to each other. They don't look the same with one of them fat and the other slim. Somehow, their bodyweight is exactly the same. How can that be? Fat tissue takes up more space than muscle tissue which is why a fat person will look bigger. A slim person will be of the same bodyweight but, instead of the fat, they will have more muscle. Muscle tissue is more dense than fat tissue and, consequentially, it's heavier than the fat tissue. The reason I'm saying this is that you shouldn't focus on your bodyweight solely during your body transformation because there are other things going on within as well. Although it's a reasonably good indicator in general, your focus should be on the overall appearance of your body.

## MUSCLE OF THE BODY

There are 640 to 850 muscles in the human body depending on how you decide to categorise a 'muscle'. These muscles can be divided into three categories: skeletal muscle, smooth muscle and cardiac muscle. The appearance of your physique depends largely on the appearance of your skeletal muscles. For example, the muscles of your back, abdomen and legs. Skeletal muscles afford you movement, mechanic work, breathing, facial expressions, speech and the ability to keep an upright posture. These are the kinds of muscles you will be working on during your body transformation. However, do keep in mind that you need to develop all forms of skeletal muscle equally. Your body works like a unit and you need to develop it as a unit as well. Picture someone that neglects to exercise their legs. As time goes by, their legs become weak compared to their upper body and it looks odd. Like the weakest member of a unit, you are only as strong as the weakest muscle in your body so be sure to develop your body in balance. Moreover, unequal body development can cause you muscle imbalances. As many as 80% of people will experience lower back pain in their lifetime and this is often caused by the afore-mentioned muscle imbalance. Thus, it is very important that you approach your body development as needed. It is a complex integrated system. Focus on all muscle groups and don't neglect any of them. You can see the main muscle groups displayed in the following picture.

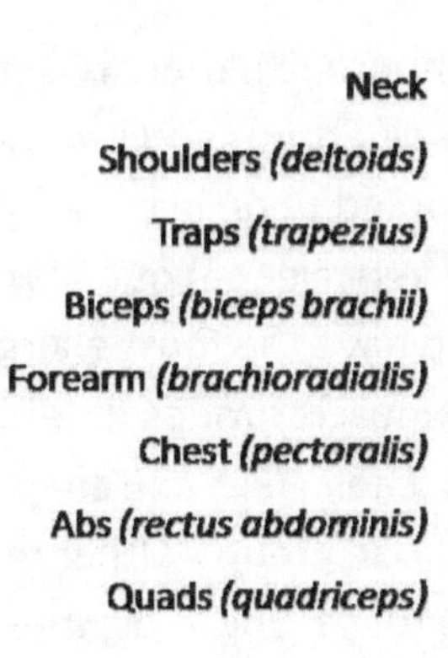
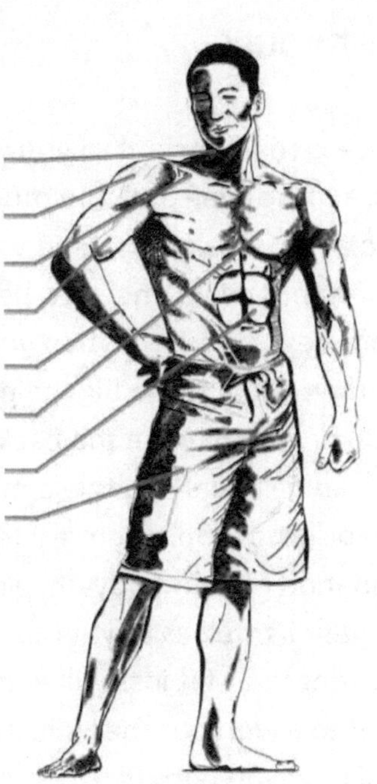

Neck
Shoulders (deltoids)
Traps (trapezius)
Biceps (biceps brachii)
Forearm (brachioradialis)
Chest (pectoralis)
Abs (rectus abdominis)
Quads (quadriceps)


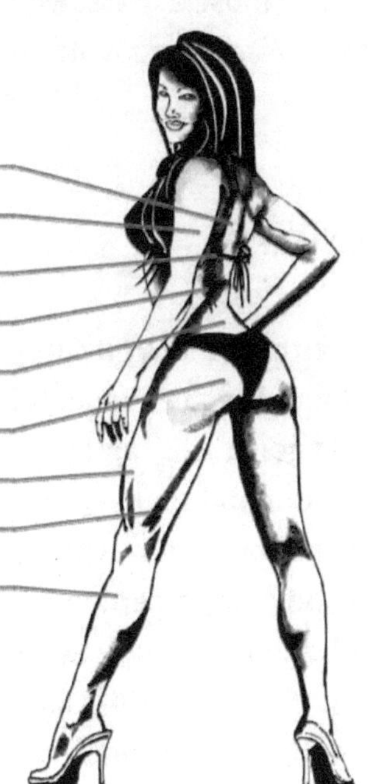

Traps (trapezius)
Triceps (triceps brachii)
Lats (latissimus dorsi)
Middle back (rhomboids)
Lower back
Glutes (gluteus maximus and medius)
Quads (quadriceps)
Hamstrings (biceps femoris)
Calves (gastrocnemius)

## MUSCLE GROUPS

As balance is so important to your approach, there is a certain procedure to working out. The muscle groups you'll work on won't be exercised all at once but instead worked upon in order. This order is very important and you need to be very clear about it. The main muscle groups are best exercised when you have the most energy and so you exercise them first. These big main muscle groups determine the shape of your body and they are the back, chest, legs and shoulders. Your focus should be mainly on these muscle groups. Other muscle groups are more or less complementary to these. These big muscle groups are the foundation of your body development. They apply to your muscle development as well as to your fat loss.  Focusing on your big muscle groups during your fat loss will engage much more muscle tissue compared to a workout that focuses on your small muscle groups. That alone will help you burn more energy. But more importantly, it will maintain your muscle mass. More lean muscle mass makes for a higher basal metabolism speed which in turn leads to greater energy use and fat loss.

## MUSCLE SHAPE

There's one thing that you can't change when it comes to your muscles and it is their ultimate shape. It is just one of those things that is determined genetically and you can't influence it. A very good example of this are your abdominal muscles. Two people can have equally well-developed abdominal muscles and they will look differently, even with the same body fat percentage. One person's muscles will have developed symmetrically, the other's non-symmetrically. Once your body fat percentage is sufficiently low and muscle mass sufficiently worked upon, you will clearly see the shape of your muscles. You'll wonder why one head of your quadriceps is particularly dominant or why is there no peak to your biceps when you're flexing. Unfortunately, this just isn't something you can change. If a particular muscle is a particular way, you won't be able to do much about it. But, if you do have a problem with a particular muscle group, try focusing on it from a different angle or work different muscle tissue that is usually less engaged by your usual exercises. Sometimes, it is enough just to change the angle of the movement and everything gets gradually corrected. Another solution for lagging muscles is their overall development as well. When you build more muscle on your body your lagging muscles will look better as well.

## RED AND WHITE MUSCLE TISSUE

The basic building units of your muscle are your muscle fibres. They can be divided into white fast-twitch and red slow-twitch fibres. They have a big influence on your workout and an understanding of the difference between them boosts both the effectiveness of your plan and your actual workout. Your muscle response to training is based on your fibre and so this is why we need to look at it. The ratio of fast-twitch and slow-twitch fibres is generally 50:50 and is again affected by your genetics. Some people have more fast-twitch fibres than slow-twitch fibres and excel in dynamic sports. On the other hand, a higher number of slow-twitch fibres makes you a perfect candidate for endurance sports. Everything comes down to the characteristics of these two types of muscle fibre. Slow-twitch muscle fibres are more efficient in constant muscle contractions during longer periods of exercise and thus endure demands longer than your fast-twitch fibres. Having a high number of these is bliss for long track runners or cyclists. Fast-twitch muscle fibres are much more efficient in fast, dynamic muscle contractions but tire much more easily which is not so great for longer workouts.
The dominance of one muscle fibre type affects what you excel at but equally, it affects the way your muscles respond to your workouts. Legs, abdominal muscles and glutes have many more slow-twitch fibres. These muscle groups will, therefore, require a somewhat different approach in your workouts. For slow-twitch groups, you will

need to do more repetitions both in your sets and exercises. It's important that this is reflected in the process of designing your workout programme.

## ADAPTABILITY TO STRESS

Your body responds to physical exertion. If you stimulate it to grow, it will grow. If you stimulate it to maintain its current state, it will do that. If you stimulate it to fat loss, it will lose some fat. It really is very simple. Think of it as learning a new language. When you learn a new language, you work with your brain and force it to adapt to your vision of how it should function. You put some effort in and expect an improvement which does come.  If you study medicine for 10 years, you become a doctor. If you play an instrument from a young age, you become an exceptional musician. When you present your brain with certain stressors, it responds appropriately. You only need to realise this simple fact and you will see the path to your new body a little more clearer. If you devote time to your body transformation, you will get the body you want and since you know already how it should look like, you only need to put some controlled effort into it.

## WHAT IS YOUR BODY NATURALLY DESIGNED FOR

The human body was primarily designed to survive in nature and it best functions when it has plenty of natural, every-day exercise as part of our day's activities. The fact that general levels of exercise and effort are vanishing from people's lives is not good. Without an ambient background level of constant body use and effort, simple tasks like lifting a heavy weight from the ground become very hard. Just think of parents that lift their babies from the ground. This activity is emulated by deadlifts in the gym. Rock climbing or tree climbing are imitated by pull ups. Your muscles have developed to be extremely functional in performing these types of activities. We used to work like this within nature and had done so for millennia. These days we need to find different ways of body development. More and more people engage in only the bare minimum of exercise during their lifetimes. People that live in big cities, in apartments and work in offices will sit all day long on their chairs. They are engaged in no physical activity during the day and the only option for them to get some decent blood circulation is to do some sports. However, if they want to get fit by introducing this better level of circulation into their muscles, it's also a good idea to develop those muscles and shape their body. That's exactly where a gym comes into play. A gym is like first aid for inactivity. Man was not designed to sit on his bottom all day long.

## TYPES OF WEIGHT LIFTING

Bodybuilding is the best activity of all for the development of your body. Nevertheless, it's not the only resistance training type by any means. Lifting can be divided into three categories: bodybuilding, powerlifting and weightlifting. The main focus of bodybuilding is body aesthetics and muscle mass building. The majority of people will encounter the basic bodybuilding principles in their gym without realising it. Bodybuilders mainly aim to build their muscle size and strength gain is more of a side effect. Bodybuilding is the exact opposite of powerlifting. Powerlifting is a sport that depends on your strength as measured by three particular exercises: benchpress, squats and deadlifts. The most important thing in powerlifting training is strength improvement and muscle volume is more or less secondary. Therefore, powerlifters train their nervous system above all. The only competitive form of lifting classified as an Olympic discipline is simply known as weightlifting, or Olympic weightlifting. The contestants compete in the snatch lift and the 'clean and jerk' lift. The key to this sport is strength and speed. Weightlifters approach their training very differently from bodybuilders and their training is not suitable for your body transformation. Body transformation utilises the principles of bodybuilding.

## BODY DEVELOPMENT

Body transformation essentially deals with fat loss and muscle building but muscle mass isn't the only thing you can work on when you're in the gym. You can also develop strength, explosiveness, speed, endurance and flexibility of your muscles. This depends on your choice of training type. As with all exercise, your body will respond and adapt to physical stress and, by working on a particular attribute, that attribute improves. However, you can't work on everything at the same time. You can only focus on one or two of those things during a workout. You can't improve everything at the same time. However, the main focus during your body transformation is your muscle mass because the appearance and ability of your body is directly connected to your muscle mass. Most deficits in things like muscle endurance or explosiveness generally won't be seen even though poor muscle flexibility can be seen in your posture straight away. Focus on getting some muscle mass built and strength will come as a by-product.

## WORKOUT METHODS

You can use a number of workout methods for your development. Circuit training, pyramids, giant sets, pre-exhaustion, negatives and many more are out there for you to discover. If you're not familiar with fitness and bodybuilding, these terms will probably be fairly new to you. You might be interested in the difference between them and wonder which method is the best to use but you don't need to. All these methods come from the basic principles of bodybuilding and you'll soon discover what these principles are. So, don't overcomplicate things and stick to the basics. They've always worked and always will because the human body ain't changing its responses any time soon. It will react always the same way when presented with these exercises.

## WOMEN AND TRAINING

Both men and women should approach their body transformation in the same way. However, for some reasons, there's this idea out there that women should approach their training differently. Some women lift ridiculously light weights and do an enormous number of repetitions. They think that this will control the shape of their muscles, despite the fact that there is nothing you can meaningfully do about that. Again, the ultimate shape of a muscle is determined genetically and can't be changed by the means of training. Not only this but female genetic muscle structure can't bulk up in the way they worry about. For all women reading this book, I have only one piece of advice that's key to an attractive physique. Women need to lift heavy weights, just like men. And by heavy, I mean weights that are relatively heavy for your ability. Push yourself to work slightly harder with heavier weights because you can't stimulate muscles growth in any other way. This won't make you bulk up too much. The idea is a fallacy and impossible for two reasons. First, women put muscle on at approximately 0.3 kilogram of lean muscle tissue per 2 months. This means the fantasy of accidentally building Schwarzenegger muscles is just not something that's going to happen. Secondly, women don't generally have the kind of hormone system designed for building an extremely muscular physique through regular exercising. If you're an exception to this, you would have already noticed it. Heavy weights are just as important for women as for men. They'll help you get a good body posture as well as that healthy and attractive physique you're looking for.

# V. Nutrition

Nutrition is probably the most important part of your body

transformation. If you don't get this right, you won't get the results you're looking for. Therefore, it's in your own interest to give this section your full attention. It includes all nutritional components that provide for the proper development and functioning of your body as well as for health maintenance. The components can be divided into two groups that are macronutrients and micronutrients. Macronutrients are protein, carbohydrates and fats and it's very important to understand them properly as muscle development and fat loss are closely connected to them. Your rate of progress depends on their quality, timing, ratio and amount. If you know how to work with them, you can influence all kinds of chemical and hormonal processes in your body. The latter affects the growth of your muscles and the storage and use of your body fat too. That's why you need to watch your daily intake of macronutrients during your body transformation. It has an enormous influence on your success.

## MACRONUTRIENTS

Let's have a closer look at particular macronutrients. Protein is a basic building material for muscle growth, even though it performs a number of other tasks depending on its content and structure. The best sources of protein are eggs, lean beef, chicken, fish, cheese and nuts. Carbohydrates, on the other hand, are a source of energy. They ce divided into simple carbs and complex carbs (also known as simple and complex sugars). Simple carbs consists of one carbohydrate building unit and are characterised by their sweet taste: examples include glucose, fructose and galactose. Your body can extract a lot of energy from them in a very short period of time. However, their overconsumption causes fat storage. Complex carbs are chains of sugars, rather than single carbohydrate units. Your body needs to dissolve them before transforming them into energy and then consequently, the energy is then released slowly. Sources of complex carbs are things like potatoes, pastries, rice and pasta. Another equally important macronutrient is nutritional fat. However, you always need to know what kind of fat you are eating as some fat is beneficial and some is detrimental. Monosaturated fat, polysaturated fat and omega-3 fatty acids are beneficial to your health. They can be found in olive oil, aubergines, peanut butter, nuts and soya. Your diet should absolutely contain these fats. On the other hand, stay away from saturated fat and transaturated fatty acids. They can be found in chicken skin, margarine, sweets and butter. This fat is detrimental to your body.

## MICRONUTRIENTS

The second nutritional group is micronutrients which are also known as vitamins and minerals. Your body can't create vitamins and minerals and so it needs to receive them from your diet. Vitamins include vitamins A, B, C, D, E and K. They're used in lots of important metabolic processes and perform many other tasks. You also need to ingest plenty of different minerals, like calcium, sodium, potassium, selenium and zinc. There are 20 minerals in total. If you've never heard of these before, that's okay. Your body only needs relatively small amounts of micronutrients and if you're eating reasonably well, you probably already receive the vitamins and minerals you need. However, be aware that a lack of micronutrients can cause you health problems. Make sure you always have enough vitamins and minerals in your diet. Strive for variety in your diet and make sure it's well balanced with lots of fruit and vegetables. That will make sure that you never have a deficit. If that does happen for any reason, you can always take the appropriate supplements.

## WHAT TO EAT

The amount of macronutrients and micronutrients that you need to eat depends on whether you want to build muscle or lose fat. The amount needed is different for both processes. Muscle building requires 2 grams of protein per 1 kilogram of your bodyweight as well as a caloric surplus. Caloric surplus is achieved by eating 5 to 9 grams of carbohydrates per 1 kilogram of your bodyweight and 0.5 to 1 gram of nutritional fat per your bodyweight. For fat loss, you still eat 2 grams of protein per 1 kilogram of your bodyweight but you create a caloric deficit. This is achieved by keeping the ratio of 0.5 to 1 gram of nutritional fat per kilogram of bodyweight in your diet and by then decreasing the amount of carbohydrates to the point where you receive 200 to 500 calories less than is needed to maintain your current bodyweight. You will discover how to get the precise number later on in the chapter so don't worry about exact calculations right now. The important thing is that you watch your macronutrient intake during your body transformation. You don't need to pay as much attention to vitamins and minerals as most peoples' diets are sufficiently varied to get these. Just make sure you have variety in your diet. Anyway, let's have a look now at how you can know the nutritional value of food and ensure you're getting what you need.


## NUTRITIONAL VALUES

In order to work out the numbers for protein, carbohydrates and fats needed for your diet, you first must learn how to use a nutrition table. This way, you get a nice overview of what particular foods consist of. A nutrition table is like a compass for your nutrition and it's fantastic for understanding what you actually eat. Nutrition tables show you the amount of protein, carbohydrates and fat in 100 grams of a given food, as well as its energy value. Some tables even show the amount of micronutrients in the foods.  By using a table, you get to know what your daily caloric intake should look like. However, don't forget that all numbers are given for 100 grams of a given food.  For working out daily intakes, you need to weigh your food and then calculate the appropriate values from the table. So, if you have some chicken breast that contain 20 grams of protein per 100 grams and your portion is 200 grams, the overall protein content of your portion will be 40 grams. Also, remember that these numbers are calculated for foods in their raw state so, if you cook some rice, don't forget to weigh it before you cook it. Cooked rice contains water so weighing rice soaked in water won't give you the right value. Learn how to use the nutrition table and make sure your food always provides you with the sufficient amount of nutrients.

## FOOD TASTE AND FUNCTION

Controlling your diet doesn't have to affect the taste of your food. The right taste and best structure for your food can easily be achieved together. If you've neglected the macronutrient contents of your food until now, it might be little harder for you at the beginning. However, it's no problem for someone who is familiar with nutritional values of food and, if you understand the basic cooking principles and work with the nutrition table, it won't cause you any problems whatsoever. You don't need to know a single recipe. If you understand basic cooking principles, you only need to choose some ingredients and prepare something edible. It doesn't need to be a work of art. As time goes on, you'll find out what you like and the taste of your food will develop by itself. However, remember that your food will serve you as an energy source as well as the material for building and recovery of your muscle fibres. The priority is the nutritional content of the foods, not the taste.

## MEAL PLANS AND CUSTOMIZATION

One of the main reasons you need to learn how to prepare food yourself is that the meal plans in magazines and online aren't designed for you. They contain the right foods but their ratios and amounts are often chaotic. These meal plans simply won't cater to your specific situation. The people that design them aren't thinking of you personally when they do so. Designing a meal plan to suit everyone doesn't even make sense. Everybody has a different bodyweight, different body composition and has a different daily energy expenditure. Make sure your meal plan considers all these things and that you tailor your meal plan for your specific needs. If you get a sufficient knowledge of your body and which foods to use in which amounts, you'll find this easy. If you're not so sure about it, I suggest you get an advice from someone who understand these things. Call your personal trainer and ask them to design a customized meal plan for you. Any personal trainer that's serious about their job should know how to design this. A proper meal plan is an important tool that will help you get the results that you want so make sure you get one that's right for you.

## RECOMMENDED DAILY ALLOWANCE (RDA)

Don't waste your time by following the recommended daily allowance guidelines. If you really want to read the food label, only look at the macronutrients. The problem with food labels is that they give information on the recommended daily allowance percentage for one eating portion which is completely misleading. So, if you eat 100 grams of cottage cheese containing 11 grams of protein per 100 grams, the information on the label will say that it represents 22% of the recommended daily allowance. By this measure, your recommended daily protein intake will be approximately 50 grams a day. These numbers assume your daily caloric intake to be about 2000 kcal. The first thing you need to remember is that your energy intake is not going to be 2000 kcal and your protein intake is not going to be 50 grams either. Your energy intake and protein intake will be different depending on your goals as well as on many other relevant factors. Typical recommended daily allowance numbers are completely irrelevant to your situation. They represent the sufficient daily intake for the majority of healthy people who don't need to physically change and they determine the amounts that are typically needed. However, this information is worthless to you. You are about to transform your body so you don't belong into this group of typical people. The recommended daily allowance simply doesn't consider human uniqueness, your physical activity level, your energy expenditure, nor the specific goals that you've set up for your body. The recommended daily allowance is just an attempt for defining one criteria for the mass of people. However, your diet needs to be based on your personal needs and that's why you need to organize it yourself.

## CALORIES

The unit used to measure amounts of energy is called a calorie. Every meal you eat is broken down into energy. A caloric surplus or deficit determines whether you create an anabolic environment in your body or a catabolic environment. This is why you need to count your calories diligently during your body transformation. If you want to build some muscle, there is no way of achieving it without creating an anabolic environment so you have to create one. To do this, the correct amount of calories is absolutely necessary which is why you need to count them properly. Fat loss works the same way. The only difference is that, instead of creating an anabolic environment, you also allow for a catabolic environment. Your daily energy intake will be lower during your fat loss and needs to be lower than your basal metabolism multiplied by the Physical Activity Factor. This last figure tells you how much energy your body needs to maintain its vital functions as well as covering all daily activities. To calculate this number, you can use a Schofield Equation detailed at the end of this book in one of the appendices. Find out how many calories you need and watch the amount of calories that you receive from your diet. You will be able to control your weight this way. However, if you're not careful and you take too many calories in, something undesirable will happen. You will gain fat rather than either losing it or gaining muscle. Therefore, weight control depends on the amount of calories in your diet, on your energy expenditure and on the ratio of the macronutrients that you receive from your diet. Whenever you prepare food, take a look into the

nutrition table to check the nutritional values and the energy value of
your whole meal.

## CALORIE IS NOT A CALORIE

Every nutritional component carries energy but not every one of them
are the same in terms of how you use this energy. Your body can utilise
more energy from 1 gram of fat than from one of protein or
carbohydrate. The thing is that 1 gram of protein and carbohydrates
provides approximately 4 calories while 1 gram of fat provides as many
as 9 calories. So if you know how much protein, carbohydrate and fat
you receive daily, you can calculate the number of calories. If your
caloric intake doesn't correspond with your goals, you can
subsequently adjust it. However, remember one very important thing:
if you eat 3000 calories a day and your diet consists mainly of
carbohydrates and fat, you won't have enough protein to repair your
muscle fibres. There are similar problems when you take in 3000
calories daily and all of them come from protein and fat only. Without
the carbohydrates, you'll struggle to source energy for your body. So,
calorie counting is a very important tool you should learn how to use.
However, don't rely on just one number that tells you how much
energy you receive from your diet. Different macronutrients perform
different tasks within your body and your diet should be well-balanced
with all 3 nutritional components. Focus on these three components
first and on their ratio in your diet. Only after that should you focus on
their amount, remembering that all calories are not made equal.

## METABOLISM

The process responsible for the conversion of nutrients into energy is
called metabolism. Metabolism allows the food you eat to be used as
energy. It works 24 hours a day and is influenced by multiple factors.
These influences may be age, health status or exercise intensity and

frequency. Importantly, one of the things that affect your metabolism is the amount of muscle that you have on your body. All these factors together affect the speed at which your metabolism converts the food into usable energy and this speed is called the metabolic rate. Your metabolic rate can be sped up or slowed down and you'll encounter lots of tips out there on how to speed it up. Increases in physical exercise, regular eating and sufficiently long periods of sleep will speed it up. On the other hand, lack of sleep, eating hard-to-digest food and skipping breakfast can slow it down. Ideally, you want to keep your metabolism relatively fast because the role of a metabolism is a breakdown of complex molecules and an assembly of the simple ones. The first process is called catabolism and the second is called anabolism. Anabolism and catabolism work at the same time because in order to build new body cells, there has to be a breakdown of other molecules too.

## ANABOLISM

In the world of fitness and bodybuilding, there is a great deal of talk about anabolism and catabolism. The reason is that, if you want to build some muscle, your job is to create an anabolic environment in your body. An anabolic environment is an environment where anabolism exceeds catabolism. Let's define anabolism. An anabolic process is one during which new organic substances or new structures are created. If there is a dominance of anabolism in your body, it can be said that you are growing. However, you need some energy for the molecule assembly during this process so we're back to the main source of the energy for your body which is your food. If you want to build some muscle, your diet has to become your highest priority. A caloric surplus is needed in order to create the anabolic environment. How big your caloric surplus is up to you. To start, try creating a surplus of 300 calories a day or so and watch your bodyweight. If it doesn't change in any way, add more calories and increase the surplus. Your muscles will only grow if they have the right conditions and a caloric surplus is one of these conditions. You just have to have the available materials to build muscle.

## CATABOLISM

The catabolic process is the opposite of the anabolic; a metabolic phase in which complex molecules are broken down into simple ones. If there is a dominance of catabolism in your body, your body doesn't have enough energy and will instead get its energy from its own storage. That's why you need to avoid a dominance of catabolism when building muscle. This is also the reason why there are various supplements available to suppress catabolism in your body. Whether you're aiming for muscle development or fat loss, you need to keep as much muscle as possible. The other thing is that, if there is a dominance of a catabolism in your body, your body will try to reclaim energy from your muscle tissue as well. The less muscle you have, the harder it is for you to keep a low body fat percentage and so muscle breakdown is not desirable for you in the long term. Remember that, whether your goal is to build some muscle or lose some fat, you should ideally avoid the long-term dominance of catabolism.

## WATER

Sufficient amounts of water is an important requirement for proper metabolic functioning. Don't forget to drink lots of water and keep your body hydrated. The importance of this doubles during your body transformation. The thing is that, the lack of water causes a decrease in your performance. Moreover, your water requirements increase during your body transformation. However, don't confuse water with soft drinks. A reasonable number of people drink enough liquids during the day but only a small percentage of them are actually drinking water. There is a big difference between drinking water and drinking soft drinks. Your body considers soft drinks to be a food since they have an energy value. If you have problems with drinking water, try tea. This is an acceptable substitute. Also, remember not to drink your water all at once. Spread your daily water intake throughout the day. Water is one of the most important things that you need to take care of during your body transformation. Make sure you drink enough water and drink more of it, rather than less.

## ALCOHOL

When mentioning water intake, I can't stay away from mentioning alcohol. There's a very simple rule that applies to alcohol and it can be said in two words. No alcohol. Easy to remember. If you're not persuaded, go out clubbing and then go to the gym the day after. You'll see how you'll feel and you will personally experience just what effects alcohol has on your body. In fact, you'll be lucky not to throw up or to leave without injury. It's so unpleasant that you'll never do it again. So, if you're serious about your body transformation, you will understand those two words and will stay home or learn to enjoy yourself another way. Alcohol simply doesn't go with body transformation and it is only an obstacle to developing your body. Moreover, if you train and then spend the night drinking, your hard work will be wasted and you will lose an enormous amount of effort. You won't be able to build on your progress and instead you'll have to take a step back and decrease your weights. However, unpleasant gym sessions aren't the only reason for being careful about alcohol. It also dissolves your liver glycogen, takes part in decreasing your ATP levels (immediate source of energy) and restricts the storage of ATP in your muscles. Furthermore, it slows down your metabolism, decreases your performance during workout and decreases the production of proteins. Alcohol can be very harmful to you. In fact, if you can't stay away from alcohol during your body transformation, you're probably not serious about it. Alcohol and a nightlife just don't go together with body transformation.

# VI. Supplementation

Are supplements worth the money and are they really beneficial for you? They absolutely are. However, be careful about how you approach them. Some of them are pointless. There are lot of supplements on the market and there is no point in buying them all. Use your money productively. If you decide to buy supplements, do some research first, decide whether you really need them and only buy them if that's truly the case. If you don't know which supplements will be most beneficial to you, this chapter will tell you. However, it is important to realise that the most important factors during your body transformation are still your training and nutrition. Do not expect supplements to do miracles. They are not going to do the work for you. They can help you only to the extent that you immerse yourself into your training and nutrition.

## LOW QUALITY FOOD

Before we go deeper into these supplementation issues, let's have a look at something rather disappointing that may affect your uptake of supplements. An enormous amount of supermarket food doesn't actually contain the nutrients they are supposed to have. The nutritional information is provided on the label but it's not always entirely true. Because of this, ordinary people may never get to know the true nutritional value of the foods they consume. If you buy a chicken, for example, it might not have the amount of omega-3 fatty acids it is supposed to have. This chicken never really got to move around because it lived in a limited space. Thus, you will not get your expected amount of omega-3 fatty acids from it. Moreover, this is roughly the same with your fruit, vegetables and grains, etc.. You don't know their growing conditions, the soil condition or the chemicals used for speeding up their growth. However, all these things affect their nutritional value. Think about that white water that you call milk. If you ever drank fresh milk, it would be clear to you that it's something different. I don't want to scare you and I don't want you to start farming animals or growing your own plants. I just want to underline the fact that, even though it might seem to you that you have enough nutrients in your diet, it might not be necessarily true and this is one of the very good reasons for using supplements. They are your insurance against the issues mentioned above.

## BENEFITS OF SUPPLEMENTATION

In general, the role of supplements is to ensure that you have enough material for building and repairing your muscle fibres and for the proper functioning of your body during increased physical exertion. That's the reason why they're used by professional athletes, amateur sportsmen and fitness and bodybuilding enthusiasts these days. They've become common practice in the sports world and they will help you with your body transformation as well. They can be divided into three groups: fat burners, growth stimulants and energy stimulants. They help you get stronger, recover quicker, build more lean muscle, improve your overall performance and maintain your proper body functioning. If you take a look at some supplement labels, you'll discover all kinds of other things they can help with as well. Manufacturers and sellers often make claims about supplements that aren't entirely believable so take them with a pinch of salt and don't believe everything written on these labels. They're often misleading so you need to be careful. Sellers like to take the advantage of beginners who don't know where to turn for proper advice. If it seems too good to be true, it probably is!

## MARKETING TRICKS

For both manufacturers and sellers, supplements are a multi-billion dollar business. The interesting thing is that they earn billions by selling products that people don't even need. Of course, there are some products that are an exception and you're going to learn about these products in a moment. But, think about how many people buy things they don't need because of marketing tricks that make them think they need these products. The sellers barely need to do anything to persuade people! They call an experienced bodybuilder and do a photoshoot. After that, you go to a shop and see the bodybuilder smiling at you from the cover of a fitness magazine with a tub of powder called "Extra Super Mega Biceps 15000" in his hand, giving the impression that he gained his muscle mass by using that particular product. The truth is that he probably gained his physique with the use of steroids. Anyway, he creates a certain illusion you are supposed to believe. Then, if you just add a questionable claim about the clinical research results, you basically have a best-selling product for the masses of people looking for a shortcut to muscle building. And that's not all. Besides product presentation itself, manufacturers and sellers do a couple of other tricks that I would rather not even mention. My point is that you shouldn't buy supplements just because there is a glamorous title on the label and a nice advertisement somewhere in a magazine. Your money can be and should be spent more wisely.

## PRODUCTS

So, which supplements are worth using? The main two are whey protein and creatine, whilst multivitamins and fish oil make a lot of sense as well. You don't need any other supplements. If you eat sufficient amounts of fish and nuts and your diet is well balanced with enough vitamins from things like fruit and vegetables, you don't even need the multivitamins and fish oil. You'll be all right with just some protein and creatine. Whey protein is protein isolated from whey. Whey starts as a liquid created during cheese and yoghurt production. It contains protein of the highest quality and so whey protein is brilliant for helping you gain strength, build lean muscle tissue and works well as a supplement for both pre- and post-workout. Creatine is equally good. It provides the energy for your muscles. Your body is well familiar with this substance. It can produce it itself and you'll find it in meat as well. When this substance reaches your muscles, it restores your ATP and helps you to improve your performance. Not only this, but it allows you to train harder and push your limits faster. Finally, it helps you build some lean muscle tissue and increases the strength of your muscles. That's why creatine has become the most successful supplement of the last two centuries. As long as you have a balanced diet with enough nutritional fat and vitamins, whey protein and creatine are the only two supplements you will need during your body transformation. However, if you find something else is missing in your diet, buy some fish oil and, where appropriate, multivitamins as well. Multivitamins will ensure sufficient amounts of micronutrients for your body and fish oil will enforce both sufficient amounts of nutritional fat and support for your hormones. It is proven that nutritional fat increases your testosterone level which is very beneficial during your body transformation.

## SUBSTANCES YOUR BODY IS FAMILIAR WITH

Regardless of whether you buy all 4 products or just the protein and creatine, all of them only contain substances that are found in your body or food already. So why do we add more to our diet? The reason you need to use supplements is to make sure you definitely have sufficient amounts of these substances in your body for the work you're doing. Let me explain, using creatine as an example. Creatine can be received from meat. However, you only get small amounts. There is just

4.5 grams of creatine in 1 kilogram of raw beef, 5 grams of creatine in 1 kilogram of raw pork and approximately 4 grams of creatine in 1 kilogram of tuna. So if you want to get 5 grams of creatine a day from your diet, you will need to eat more than 1 kilogram of raw meat. This is a bit of a problem. You don't eat your food raw and you always heat it during the preparation. The problem is that heat causes a breakdown of the creatine in the meat and so the amount received from your diet shrinks. This is why you should supplement creatine during your body transformation. Instead of eating an enormous amount of raw meat, you can get the exact amount of creatine that you can best utilise. It works almost the same with other supplements. The only difference is that other substances are found in your food in sufficient amounts so the biggest reason for supplementing them is their quality and usability as in the case of whey protein.


## USE AND INSTRUCTIONS


Now that you know the supplements you need, you must be wondering as to the amounts they should be taken in. Fortunately, I have the amounts and timing here for you! Let's start with creatine. When you're using creatine, make sure you ingest 5 grams a day and always use it with some quick sugars. The most convenient time for its use is immediately after your workout. Don't forget to add around 10 to 20 grams of glucose or drink a glass of fruit juice with it. Research has shown that creatine can only get to your muscles with the help of insulin which is injected into your bloodstream after you ingest glucose or some other form of quick carbs. As for whey protein, the best time to use this is both before and after your workout. You need to get nutrients into your body before your workout so you don't dip into your muscle stores for the energy. Whey protein is designed to provide you with that. You will get the nutrients in a very short time and you will be able to use them straight away. The second dose of whey protein is taken after your workout. You will be tired and you will need to top up your nutrients as soon as possible. Whey protein is very important to take at this point. For both doses, give yourself one 20-gram scoop of whey protein. Mix it into water or milk and drink it. As for multivitamins and fish oil, these can be taken when you wake up. Timing doesn't play a role with these two. However, if you use them in the morning, it's generally better as you won't have to think about them all day long. Instructions regarding amounts for these two can be found on the label of the supplement bottle itself. For a better understanding of how to use supplements, take a look now at the appendix at the end of this book.

## SUPPLEMENT BRANDS

So, now that you know the supplements you need for your body transformation, you only need to buy them. However, this is where you encounter another challenge. What brand should you choose? There are hundreds of brands these days and when you go to buy one, you may get the impression that this number is never-ending. So, how do you know what to buy when you've never done it before? The wide variety of proteins on the market can surprise you. You see, everybody has different criteria for buying supplements. Some make the decision based on their budget, some opinions will be based on recommendations, some according to their mood and lots of people want to buy everything even though they don't really know why. If you really don't know what brand to choose, get advice from someone who tried multiple brands. If you don't know anybody like that, search online. Lots of people happily share their experiences online. If you still can't decide, even after doing that, don't over-think it; simply try some out. If you find out that you don't like those ones for whatever reason, just choose something different. Otherwise, assuming you're happy with the results you're getting, just stay with the ones you chose at random.

## SUPPLEMENTATION DIFFERENCE

If you have proper training, proper nutrition and take supplements too, not only will you see the difference swiftly but it will be enormous too. If we look at two people training for one year under the same conditions with one taking supplements and the other one not, the person who takes supplements will get their desired results much faster than the person who doesn't take supplements. If they both work out for one year, the difference might even be noticeable within a couple of months. Supplements accelerate the process of your body transformation. But you need to know exactly what you're doing and, again, the best thing that you can do for yourself is to invest some time into acquiring some knowledge about how supplements really work. If you're going to use them, it's also important that you take time to know what is going to happen to your body.

# Part 3
# Muscle Gain

# VII. Muscle Gain Philosophy

Although resistance training is key to your muscle development, lots of people still avoid going to the gym. Is it possible to build muscle without going to the gym? Yes, it is. However, there is a limit on how much muscle you can build and it will only continue for a certain amount of time before the gains stop. If you start doing exercises like push ups or lunges, you will be able to stimulate your muscles for a while. You'll force them to grow and you'll be able to apply the principle of 'progressive overload' as well. Progressive overload keeps your workouts demanding and makes sure they are always effective. However, you will get to a point when your muscles stop growing and your workouts will have met their upper limits for strength and endurance development. The resistance you need to overcome will become insufficient for further improvement, thwarting this strategy. This is a problem as the principle of progressive overload is critical to your muscle development and it's necessary to include it in your training philosophy. This is why you shouldn't look for a way to build your muscle without lifting weights. These methods eventually limit themselves. Instead, using weights allows you to apply the principle of progressive overload over a sustained period of time. Whenever it gets too easy, just use a heavier weight or add a couple of plates to your bar and your workout is equally demanding again.

## PROGRESSIVE OVERLOAD

If you want to get bigger, you need to get stronger as well. Your muscles always adapt to your workload and so if you want to stimulate them sufficiently, you need to constantly bombard them with heavier weights. That's why you should strive for improvement every time you're in the gym and beat your performance from your last workout. Although, this isn't always possible, you still need to try. Progressive overload is the basic principle of bodybuilding. Every time your body adapts to the weights you lift, you need to increase the weight of your resistance. Your body won't change without some kind of stimulus and you need to force it to see the need for change. The whole process is very similar to climbing a ladder. If you're not increasing your weights, you are staying on the same 'ladder step' without moving up. However, if you increase the weight of your resistance, you're moving one step upwards at a time. If you can do more than 12 reps in one set, add more weight to your particular exercise. Increase your weight and then carry out the exercise until you've worked your way back to the same number of reps. If you were able to do 10 reps before, expect to do maybe 7 reps next time. Whilst the heavier weight is a new challenge for you and your muscles, your next goal is to always try to get to a level where you can do 12 reps again, thus allowing you to increase the weight again as well. Increasing the weight of your resistance is central to your muscle development. If you want to build some muscle, always try to lift heavier weights each and every workout. This is the principle of progressive overload.

## BASIC WORKOUT FOR THE BEGINNERS

When you're building muscle, stick to the basics. Train regularly, train smart, train hard, lift heavy and increase your weights. Start with the basics and stay with them from beginning to end. Lot of people think that the basic workout you'll use is for beginners only. They think that there are more effective or 'special' exercises for more experienced bodybuilders. They learn the basics, work on themselves, see the first results and then they start speculating. They swap those effective exercises they're using for other exercises, just because someone else is doing them. They see them in a magazine next to those pictures of the buff models or in the gym and automatically link them with the higher level of success. However, those exercises, whilst technically more advanced, might not be that much more effective for your muscle development and that's the important thing that these people don't know. They either think they are really more effective or they just want to show off and be like the experienced bodybuilders. Don't do this. If there's something that works for you, there is no reason for you to change it. You only need to stick to the basics and gradually increase the weight. You will build your body up.

## BUILD SOME BACKGROUND BEFORE GOING FOR MUSCLE GAIN

While you're waiting to get started on your journey, make sure that you prepare for everything that's coming up. You will invest a lot of time and energy into muscle building and it would be a shame to waste it just because you're not prepared for shortcomings here and there. Make sure you use your time and energy to the best of your ability and prepare for your muscle development. If you've never been to a gym or have no idea how your diet should look, starting your journey won't be easy and you mustn't expect to get your results immediately. You're not going to build your body overnight. First, focus on the basic things and then develop the other stuff gradually. It's like building a house. You got to have a good foundation because, otherwise, it's only a question of time as to when it will fall apart. Focus on the basics, learn how to design a workout programme and understand how to perform your exercises correctly. You do it for both your success and your security. Your knowledge will save you from discovering that, instead of putting on two kilograms during the first two weeks, you've actually lost them from eating incorrectly or working out more than your diet allows. Also, you'll save yourself from various injuries that could interrupt your transformation. So, take time to build some background in the gym before embarking on your journey.

## THE FASTEST TRACK OF PROGRESS

If there's anything you don't understand, always ask. Ask experienced people and listen to what they say. Their advice will help you to avoid mistakes that are easily made at the beginning. Ask your personal trainer and the people around you that are making the fastest progress. However, do not automatically ask the biggest guy or the girl with the most attractive body. The biggest guy might be the biggest because he's using banned substances and the girl could have been a gymnast from a very young age, making her body unobtainable for the vast majority of people. Although they have perfect bodies and lots of knowledge, they might not had to go through what you want to go through. Instead, you need to get advice from someone who has gone through what you want to go through which is a body transformation. Thus, the best advice you can get is from someone who started where you are now and worked their way to where you want to be. You can also get fantastic advice from whoever's progressing the fastest in the gym. But again, do make sure their speed of progress isn't based on banned substances.

## EQUALITY

Good looking people should inspire you. The only thing you need to realize about them is that, at some point, they probably started exactly where you are right now and, if you'd started working out at the same time as them, you could look just as good now. So, look to them as your inspiration. Although they might look better than you right now, you're all equal in the gym when you're doing your workouts. After all, you're putting the same effort and quality in. The only difference is that these people have been doing it longer than you and that can't be overlooked at this point. Ignore the fact that someone can lift 100 kilograms on a benchpress while you lift 50 kilograms. Fitness and bodybuilding are not about how much you lift. Fitness and bodybuilding are about contracting your muscles and pumping the blood to them whilst you're enjoying the pump. It's about whether you can adequately stimulate your muscles for growth. The weight that you lift is only a tool that you use so don't be intimidated by people that lift more than you. They deserve some respect, of course but the important thing to focus on is what they're doing for their body today and you too can do the same.

## YOUR CONFIDENCE AND YOUR CHARACTER

One day, when you get to the point when you become the inspiration for others, it is very important that you keep your feet firmly on the ground. The thing is that your confidence will probably grow as your body gets more attractive. However, take care not to be cocky or arrogant. An attractive body doesn't make you someone more important or special than everyone else. Your muscular or slim body can give you a feeling of power but that doesn't mean you should exercise it over others to behave superior. Stay human. Your body transformation is supposed to hone your character, not deteriorate it. It develops your discipline, fairness, responsibility, reliability, perseverance, precision and many other positive personality traits. You'll develop a range of personality traits you can appreciate in yourself as well in others you meet every day. Embody these qualities and don't get caught up in acting out a petty superiority complex.

## A WORKOUT PROGRAMME

Let's get back to your muscle development. Your goal is to have sufficient knowledge to design your workout programme yourself. Don't rely on other workout plans and design one yourself. Then compare it with other trustworthy plans you come across and adjust it as appropriate. The thing is that, if you don't have sufficient knowledge to design your workout plan, you can't feel confident in the plan you do choose. This is why the next chapter provides you with some important points about designing your plan. Learn as much as you can and if you're still not confident about what you're sure of, get some advice. Hire a personal trainer. Tell them what your personal goals are and what your ordinary day looks like and they'll explain how to design a personal workout plan for you. Ask them about the reason for using the exercises they're using, why do you need to do a particular number of sets and reps and why they set up the rest interval as it is. Every good personal trainer will teach you about these things because they're interested in having you understand them. If you understand these things, it increases your chances for success enormously. If you understand the basic stuff, you will also be able to understand other details as well, whether you find them in books, magazines or online. Having this initial knowledge will help you move forward much quicker.

## THE BEGINNERS SUPER SPEED

So, once you're ready to build some muscle, just make the first step. Although the beginning might be hard for you, your progress will be massive. You see, new types of impulse shock your body the most. And what does your body do in response? It adapts proportionately. That's why beginners whose bodies are least used to this type of physical exercise always experience the best progress. It's because lifting is completely unfamiliar to their body. So, if you are a beginner too, your initial results will probably shock you. Never again will you experience the same rate of progress as at the beginning of your body transformation. The longer you work out after that and the closer you are to fulfilling your genetic potential, the slower your progress will be. Both your muscle building and your fat loss will slow. The thing is that, no matter how much you want to build more muscle or lose more fat, it can't go on forever. It simply has to stop somewhere. That's why people that are approaching their genetic potential gloriously celebrate every kilogram of a lean muscle tissue built or every decimal place shrunk from their body fat percentage.


## WITH EVERY MISTAKE THERE COMES A LESSON

You're always going to make a couple of mistakes during your body transformation. Even with maximum knowledge about your training, nutrition and supplementation, it'll happen. It's because we are human, not robots. The important thing to realize is that the process of learning brings valuable mistakes with it so don't look at them negatively. When you were a child, you didn't do everything perfectly at the first time. You fell down when you were learning how to walk and you made all kinds of funny sentences when you were learning to talk. Mistakes don't keep you behind on your path. Instead, every mistake offers you a lesson. Every fall you had when walking taught you how to do it better next time and every 'I go-ed home' brought you closer to talking. In other words, with every mistake you make, look for the lesson behind it. The majority of people consider mistakes to be something bad because that's what they've been taught. However, the truth is that you learn more from your mistakes than anything else so don't allow yourself to be discouraged by them. Always look for the positive side and remember that you're not failing, you're *learning*. It is better to strive for success and make mistakes than to let the fear of failure to keep you from working on your dreams.

## HOW TO APPLY THE TRANSFORMATION ROCKET

The Transformation Rocket will help you to avoid some mistakes too. Let's have a look at how it does that.

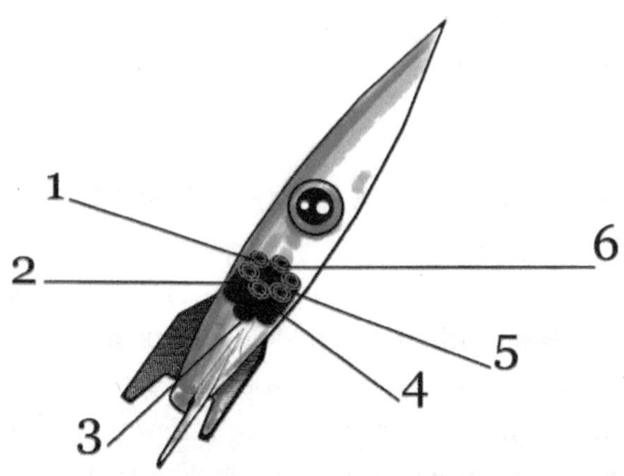



*1. Decision 2. Discipline 3. Time 4. Training 5. Nutrition 6. Supplementation*

1. Decision – If you really want to build some muscle, you need to work on it systematically. However, that requires you deciding to invest time into your body transformation and to approach it seriously. You have to decide to choose the gym instead of clubbing, water over alcohol and a proper amount of sleep rather than TV.

2. Discipline – If you devote 10 hours a day to your body transformation but have no discipline during the rest of the day, your body will recognise it and won't develop. That's why you need to put some discipline into the whole process; your body is sharp and will notice otherwise. Work out when you're supposed to work out, get quality food in the right amount tand maintain a healthy lifestyle. Do it 24 hours a day and do it all throughout your programme.

3. Time – After the first week, you might seem a bit bigger already. However, don't think you've gained actual muscle. Your muscles are actually swollen by glycogen and water due to your increased nutrition intake. You'll have to train longer to see some real muscle growth. So, be patient and don't slack at the first hint of success because it is going to take some time.

4. Training – Make sure your workouts are intense and difficult enough. Use mainly compound exercises as described in the upcoming chapter, stay within a 6 to 12 rep range and keep applying the principle of progressive overload. You really need to stimulate your muscles consistently so that they get the signal to grow. However, be careful not to exercise too much. 20 sets for a muscle group during one workout won't achieve anything.

5. Nutrition – Make sure you create a caloric surplus every day and receive approximately 2 grams of protein for 1 kilogram of your bodyweight. Eat enough protein, carbohydrates and fat as all 3 macronutrients are very important. Spread your food all throughout the day and make sure that at least 80% of your diet consists of very high-quality food.

6. Supplementation – Whey protein, creatine, multivitamins and fish oil will all help you build bigger and stronger muscle. If you want to maximize the results of your muscle gain, use all four. However, if you don't want to use all four of them, make sure you include at least whey protein and creatine.

# VIII. Muscle Gain Workout Structure

When it comes to your muscle development, there are two

fundamental approaches that you can choose. These are a fullbody workout and a workout split. The majority of rules about to be mentioned in this chapter apply to both of the approaches. However, some are different so let's have a look at the characteristics of both of these approaches. A fullbody workout is a workout in which you work all your muscle groups on the same day. On the other hand, there's the workout split where you train individual muscle groups on different days. Each approach has its own advantages and it doesn't matter which one you choose at the beginning. Both of them will help you build some muscle. Your muscles are not used to exercising and they will react to anything. When you later develop a certain level of muscle mass, you can change your approach and compare which is more effective for you. If you start with a workout split, try changing to a fullbody workout after a couple of months. Or, if you start with a fullbody workout, experiment with a workout split. Find out what works best for you and stick to it. That's what it's all about, after all. You have to find what's best for you and what helps you to build muscle more effectively. Some people get better results from one and some from the other. If you've been using the fullbody approach and you then find a personal trainer that prefers a workout split, give it a try. If they've decided that it's best for you, trust them. If you need to decide on your own and you don't know which approach to choose, pick one and use it for a couple of months. Just don't think about changing it every few days.


## BIG MUSCLE GROUPS

Regardless of whether you choose a fullbody workout or a workout split, your focus should be primarily on your big muscle groups. That is, your back, chest, shoulders and legs. It applies to both your overall body development as well as to the exercise order of your workout. Big muscle groups are the muscle groups that determine the appearance of your body so, to get the shape you're going for, it's important that they're what you focus on the most. You should always use the classic compound exercises when you're training your big muscle groups. If you're afraid that you're not going to work your smaller muscle groups enough this way, don't worry. There's room for your smaller muscle groups' development and isolated exercises within both types of workout. However, remember to keep to the right order when performing your exercises. If you want to concentrate on a combination of bigger and smaller muscle groups, always work your big muscle groups first. This is because you'll have the most energy at the beginning of your workout and so you can exploit it best by working your big muscle groups first. At the end of the day, these are the muscle groups that matter the most when it comes to the appearance of your physique. Smaller muscle groups are only a complement to those big ones.

## COMPOUND AND ISOLATION EXERCISES

The base of all workouts are always compound exercises. Compound exercises are multi-joint exercises that work multiple muscles at the same time. Good examples of these are back squats, deadlifts or benchpress. However, there are also some isolation exercises that work just one muscle or muscle group only. During isolation exercises, you basically perform a single joint movement. An example of such an exercise is a leg curl. Compound exercises are useful as they are far more effective than isolation exercises. Therefore, your job during your body transformation is to use mainly compound exercises that can be supported by isolation exercises as appropriate. Compound exercises allow you to use heavy weights that stimulate your muscle and strength growth the most and you also engage far more muscle fibres. That's why if you choose to do a fullbody workout, almost all of your exercises will be compound exercises. On the other hand, if you're doing a workout split, make sure that at least two out of three exercises are compound exercises and that you use a weight heavy enough to get into that 6 to 12 rep range. Your physique will start to grow in size because compound movements are very demanding. They allow you to work hard and, your body will have to react to that. However, always ensure that you do them properly. You're working with heavy weights and safety comes always first.


## HOW TO CHOOSE YOUR EXERCISES

So, let's have a look at which exercises are compound exercises. The following list details the exact exercises you will use the most in your workouts:


<u>Chest:</u> benchpress with a barbell or dumbbells, incline or decline benchpress with a barbell or dumbbells and dips;
<u>Back:</u> deadlifts, undergrip pull ups, overgrip pullups, lat pulldowns, seated cable rows, bent-over rows, one-arm dumbbell rows, T-bar rows, various further types of rows;
<u>Legs:</u> squats and their variations, deadlifts and their variations, leg press, lunges;
<u>Shoulders:</u> military press, shoulder press with a barbell, dumbbells or on a smith machine, upright row;
<u>Biceps:</u> undergrip pull ups and various undergrip pulling exercises;
<u>Triceps:</u> dips and close grip benchpress.

If you've never done these exercises, it pays to watch some videos that explain how to do them properly. However, if you're totally new to the gym, hire a personal trainer and they will introduce you to all these exercises as standard.


## WORKOUT FREQUENCY

If you know what exercises are the most effective for you, let's look at how to design your workout programme. First, we should think about how often you'll train because this affects how quickly your muscles can recover. Your muscles can only grow properly if you give them enough time for recovery. This time is different for everyone and depends on your diet, proper sleep and rest too. One person can recover in two days and work the same muscles again on the third day and another person might need three to four days for their recovery. It's very individual and that's why your job is to find out how much time you need for your recovery. Find out how many days you need and adjust your plan according to your findings. One thing to remember though is not to exercise the same muscle group every day. If you work the same muscle group every day, you won't gain any muscle as a consequence. Lots of people train their abs this way even though abdominal muscles are no different from the other muscle groups and require the same approach. If you work your legs, back and shoulder twice a week, then only work your abs twice a week as well and always do only three to four exercises with 3 sets of each. Do 15 reps in a set and if that's too easy for you, use weights too. If you want to develop your abdominal muscles, then treat them the same way as your hamstrings or quadriceps. Stick to this advice and you'll get your six-pack very soon. However, if you ignore it and work your abs every day, they won't grow because they will be tired. Instead, you will use up all the energy needed for growth and you will get flat abs with no size. So, remember not to work any muscle group each and every day. At best, you won't make progress and in the worst case scenario, you will actually lose some muscle mass. Your muscles must have sufficient time for recovery. Let's say you do a three day split, for example. Day one is a push day, so you exercise your chest, shoulders and triceps. On day two, you do some pulling exercises, which means you work your back and biceps and day three is a leg day. Your job is to find out how much time each group needs for recovery. Are you going to work out three days in a row and then take a day off? Will you take two days off? Will you train every other day? The time you need for your recovery is highly individual and something you need to find out yourself. Don't forget that if you do fullbody workouts, the demand on the various groups is lower and so your muscles can recover quicker as a result. In that case, you can work the same muscle group as much as three times a week. However, the demand is higher when doing a workout split and so you can only train the same muscle group every 3 to 5 days.


## WORKOUT PLANNING

When you find out how long it takes you to recover and how often can you actually go to the gym, you can start planning what to do in the gym. Decide which muscle groups are you going to work on. How long will your rest intervals be? How many different exercises and how many sets for each will you do? Everything should be planned in advance. You should even know the weight you'll be lifting for each exercise. However, don't plan too far ahead. You don't know whether you'll be able to lift 10 pounds more in 2 weeks or not. Plan one day in advance. If this process isn't automatic and easily memorable for you, write it down. The main point here is that you need to have your workout designed in advance so you don't spend ages wandering around the gym trying to figure out what to do next. An ideal workout is when you enter the gym, know exactly why you went there, work exactly what you need to and then leave. No brainstorming, no creativity, no discussions. This kind of approach will enable you to concentrate on yourself and on every single rep in your workout.


## WORKOUT DURATION

If you choose to do a workout split, you will typically spend about 50 to 60 minutes in the gym including your warm-up and post-workout stretching. You will do about 18 sets in total, which takes about 45 minutes to do. Don't do 30 sets just because you've seen it in some magazine. Your body won't be able to recover properly before hitting the gym again if you do 30 sets. With natural bodybuilding, your hormones can sustain only a certain level of workload so don't overdo it. Of course, everybody's different and if you find out you can do 20 sets in a workout and still grow, then do 20 sets if you want. Observe your body and find out what it responds to best. A fullbody workout is a bit different when it comes to these things. With fullbody workouts, you can easily do 20 or more sets as it's spread between all your muscle groups. Besides, you get a day off after every workout so your body will be able to recover despite the workload. However, even if you find yourself able to do 20 sets, still try to keep your workouts as brief and as intensive as possible. One of the reasons for this is the release of catabolic hormones which you need to avoid. Quick and intensive workouts are your protection against an excessive release of cortisol. Cortisol is a catabolic hormone that slows down proteosynthesis and creates a negative nitrogen balance within your body. That means that more protein is broken down than is synthesized. There are some positive things about cortisol as well but from the point of view of bodybuilding, the negatives are more important and so you need to avoid introducing excessive amounts of this hormone. A short and intensive workout is one way of accomplishing this.

## NUMBER OF SETS

Fullbody workouts allow you to do more sets then workout splits. However, the load on your individual muscle groups is lower. You'll do only 3 to 5 sets per muscle group depending on how your fullbody workout is designed. It all depends on how you design your workouts and how many reps are you doing in a set. Sometimes, you can do 18 sets in a workout and sometimes as many as 25. However, the total rep count for a muscle group stays roughly the same at all times. A workout split is very different in this respect. With a workout split, you focus on one, two or three muscle groups only and you do about 7 to 9 sets for each of them. For the big muscle groups, you do 8 to 9 sets and for the small ones, you do 7 to 8 sets. Those 8 or 9 sets for big muscle groups can be divided into 3 exercises of 3 sets or into 2 exercises of 4 sets.

Smaller muscle groups can be divided into 3 exercises again, with the first two exercises involving 3 sets and the third, 2 sets. So, if you work your chest and triceps on the same day, it'll look something like this. You start with your chest by doing 3 exercises of 3 sets which totals 9 sets and then you continue with 2 exercises of 3 sets and 1 exercise of 2 sets for your triceps which totals 8 sets. In total, you do 17 sets. Simple maths. This will be enough to stimulate your muscles but at the same time, you won't overdo it. Remember that, if you do overdo it, you'll likely strip yourself of the energy needed for muscle growth.

## FIXED REP COUNT AND REP RANGE

Whilst it's important to have a routine that you've carefully thought about, don't limit yourself to a particular rep count as it's unnecessary. The thing is that, if you set yourself up for 3 sets with 8 reps in each, you won't try to push beyond that. You'll do 8 reps and stop because you've 'finished'. You might be capable of doing 9 or 10 reps and you could instead be pushing your limits further which would then force your muscles to grow again. That's why you should avoid a fixed rep count. Another problem is that you need a longer rest between your sets. Longer rests means your workout is longer as well and you already know the issues with a long workout. Instead of a fixed rep count, try to work in a rep range. The ideal rep range for stimulating the muscle growth is 6 to 12 reps. When you're working your legs and abs, this rep range goes up to 12 to 20 reps. This is because there are more slow-twitch muscle fibres in these muscles. So, if you work within a rep range instead of using a fixed rep count, you'll be able to push yourself to do as many reps as you can. Imagine doing a shoulder press. Instead of doing 3 sets of 10, you do 3 sets of 6 to 12 with the same weight. In your first set, you could manage 11 reps, in your second set10 and in your third set, just 8. You do as many reps as you can in each set. If you did 3 sets of 10 reps, you wouldn't have been able to push your limits in the first set. Smaller rest intervals will make sure your workout intensity is high enough and will shorten your time spent in the gym. Not only that but in each of those 3 sets, there are enough reps for stimulating muscle growth and so you provide your muscles with the perfect workout. So remember that a rep range gives you more opportunity than a fixed count. The only thing you need to do is to choose a weight that will allow you to do no more than 12 reps.

## ADEQUATE WEIGHTS

Light weights don't really help you with building your muscle that much. If you can do 25 reps in a set, your weights are far too light and instead of working on your muscle size, you start working on your muscle strength and muscle endurance. That's why you should always choose to work with heavy weights. However, don't overdo it again. Weights that are too heavy will not help you with your muscle development either. If you can do only 1 to 5 reps with a particular weight, you will only develop your strength again. If you think you can do 8 reps with such weight anyway, forget it. Lot of people focus on lifting as heavy as they can and they forget to keep proper form while doing it. They don't control the weights, use the momentum, use the cheating technique and generally struggle. So, first of all, always use weights you are able to control. It's always better to work with lighter weights and to use a proper exercise form than to work with heavier weights and either be unable to engage your muscles properly or expose yourself to danger by using a poor exercise form. Don't listen to your ego when you're choosing your weights. You're not in the gym to show other people that you can lift heavy. You're there to exercise your muscles. Leave your ego at the door.

## HEAVY WEIGHTS

Heavy weights are significant in developing muscle. If you simply want to get bigger, you also need to get stronger and you will get stronger by lifting heavy weights. Working with heavy weights sends your muscles a clear signal to grow. Your muscles will simply have to grow to prepare in case you expose them to the same workload again. And that's exactly what you'll do. But, don't labour under a misapprehension about heaviness. 'Heavy weight' doesn't mean lifting 150 kilograms during benchpress or something like that. Heavy weights are the weights that are heavy enough for you. If 70 kilograms is heavy enough for your benchpress and you can fatigue your muscles or finish 1 or 2 reps before fatiguing your muscles (while staying in that 6 to 12 rep range), use this weight. When this weight ceases to be demanding for you, you will raise it. That is the principle of progressive overload you've read about in a previous chapter. Remember that you need to control the weights you choose. It's not enough just to mechanically lift it. You need to control both phases of your lift. You need to control both the positive and negative phase of the lift. If you stick to this advice, you shouldn't expose your joints to danger.


## WORK UNTIL FAILURE


In any given set, try to do as many reps as you can. Working to failure is a very good technique for getting your results. Failure is when you can't do another rep while keeping a proper exercise form. So if you do 7 bicep curls, feel you could do one more and just manage it, it's a repetition that you reached failure with. I guarantee you, you could do more reps but your exercise form would be very poor in that case, negating the useful effects of the set. So work until failure or finish one or two reps before you reach the failure. It still stimulates your muscles sufficiently. When you complete reps that start to hurt, your body receives a signal that it needs to grow because you're going to bombard it with the same workload next time.  This makes it get ready for this kind of situation and grow more muscle. If you're not sure about whether to work until failure or to finish one or two reps before failure, you have the same choice as before. Choose the one you like, try it out and, if you need to, change to the other. Sometimes work to failure and sometimes finish one rep before failure. Some gets results from the former and some from the latter. Just keep in mind that your training needs to be always challenging for you. Observe how your body reacts to both options and you will find out what works best for you.

## REST INTERVALS

The rest interval between your sets should be long enough for your muscles to recover but not too long for your blood to leave your muscles. That's why a lot of personal trainers recommend a rest interval of 1 to 2 minutes, which is fairly suitable for beginners. Exercising is a bit of a shock for their muscles so, if you're just starting on your journey, stick to this rest interval too. However, if you've already been working out for some time, start with a rest interval of 45 to 60 seconds. Shorter breaks will enforce a higher workout intensity and because you're more experienced, you don't need to worry about not being able to sustain it. You can probably achieve about 12 reps in your first set, 10 reps in your second set and 8 reps in your last set. If you've no problem with completing more than 6 reps in your last set, there's no reason to have breaks that are longer than 45-60 seconds. Moreover, your performance will by affected by the creatine as well. If you use it during your body transformation, you'll find it easy to complete enough reps while keeping the short rest intervals. If 45 to 60 seconds isn't enough for you and you feel you need more time for rest between your sets, just take more rest. Gradually increase your rest interval up to 2 minutes, allowing yourself 10 seconds more per set. However, if you find you can exercise with shorter breaks, stick to them and experiment with cutting them down to 30 seconds but not less. It will help you increase your workout intensity which is very important for your muscle development. Moreover, you will finish your workout relatively quickly which will help to avoid the excessive amounts of catabolic hormones in your body.

## MOVEMENT SPEED

Lot of beginners do their reps too fast. They completely neglect the negative phase of the movement and cheat by using momentum during the positive phase of the movement. The best example of this is the benchpress. They put the plates on and start lifting. They lower the barbell to their chest, bounce it for at least a third of the movement and push the other two-thirds. They're not really engaging their muscles during the lowering phase and, thanks to the bouncing motion, they only engage them partially during the pushing movement itself. This is no way to develop your muscles. To avoid it, you need to choose a speed that is optimal for you when lifting your weights. Make sure you can control the weights with the muscles you are working on and that you can control them in every moment of the movement. If you can't control the movement, decrease the weight. Too-heavy weights are one of the main reasons that people use improper lifting tempo. They don't control the weights they choose. Remember to choose the proper weight and don't try to complete a couple of additional awkward reps. Completing one additional rep with disastrous exercise form isn't going to help anyway. Remember that lifting is not about how many reps you can do. It's about contracting your muscles and giving them a proper workout. If you exercise with a reasonable tempo and control your weights fully, you'll soon be on your way to seeing some growth in your muscles. Don't swing, don't use momentum and don't cheat. It's better to decrease your weights and work your way back up.

## EXERCISE FORM

Besides a proper lifting tempo, focus on achieving the proper exercise form. Proper exercise form ensures that you work your muscles properly and minimize the risk of injury at the same time. Lots of people experience difficulties with their exercise form even after they've been working out for a while. During your benchpress, for example, a grip that is too wide or positioned badly transfers the tension from your chest to your shoulders. As a consequence, your pectoral muscles perform an insufficient amount of work and aren't stimulated enough for growth. Moreover, you're exposing yourself to a shoulder injury. Other examples could be bent-over rows and overall back development. If you're using weights that are too heavy and your muscle-mind connection is weak on top of that, the chances are that, instead of working your back, you're working your arms. Although you're doing 'back' exercises, the resistance is being lifted via a massive engagement of your arms. As a result, your back muscles are not stimulated enough for growth. When it comes to training your back and chest muscles, remember that your arms serve as hooks that connect your body to the weights you're lifting. Remember that the trajectory of the movement is only performed by your elbows and not by the entire arm. That's how you overcome the resistance with the muscle groups you are trying to work on at the moment. If you don't feel the pump or you don't feel a proper level of fatigue in the muscles you were supposed to be working on, it's high time you thought about the exercise form of the exercises you're doing. Always work with the muscles you're supposed to work with and only go to the point where you can still feel tension in your muscles. If the tension leaves or suddenly gets better at the top of the lift, you've likely locked your joints.  This is a problem as it means your muscles can't develop further as they aren't actually being worked.


## MACHINES AND THEIR USE


There is plenty of debate about which is better for your muscle development: free weights or machines? Some praise the former and some the latter. However, all opinions are subjective. Let's go for reason instead. There are a couple of facts you can rely on. Free weights engage your stabilising muscles more than machines. On the other hand, machines offer you greater safety during your workout. So, if you're trying to build some muscle and you're not a professional athlete with highly specific goals, you can choose either of them. Professional athletes will benefit more from using the free weights because of the benefit to their stabilising muscles. However, what matters during your body transformation is only whether your muscles grow. In that case, both free weights and machines are suitable for you. If you can get the blood flowing into your muscles properly with the use of machines, feel free to use them. They can be a very good asset to your workouts. Moreover, the best machines for your workouts are mainly unilateral machines, that is, machines that only use one limb at a time, rather than the pair. Anyway, both free weights and machines have something to offer. Combine them in your workouts and you will be able to push your limits even further.

## NEED FOR CHANGE

When you decide on your approach to your resistance training, stick to it. Regardless of whether you choose to use free weights or machines, a workout split or a fullbody workout or whether you work out 3 days or 4 days a week, just pick one combination and stick to it. Try to get the most out of it whilst you can because your body will gradually get used to it and after some time, it will stop responding to your workouts. This is called 'hitting a plateau'. When you keep working out but your bodyweight and strength stop increasing, it's time for you to change something in your workouts. You don't need to change your workout entirely, but something certainly needs altering. What is often needed is just changing one or two exercises, changing the exercise order or switching from a barbell to dumbbells. The change doesn't have to be massive. You only need a little tweak. Your body will notice the change and start responding to your workout with further growth designed to counteract your new movements. If you're asking whether you need to tweak your workouts regularly, the answer is no. If you're gaining muscle, you don't need to change anything. If you're getting results from your current workouts, carry on with it and only change it when you start plateauing. There's no reason for change if things are working as they're supposed to. Some people might like prevention and so they change something in their workout more frequently but if you change things too often, it's not too good for you either. The thing is that, if you keep changing your exercises every week, you're not going to be able to apply the principle of progressive overload enough. You can't increase a weight if you stopped using it in an exercise last week so stick to your training until it stops bringing you the results. Little tweaks, when appropriate, will help you to maximize the response of your body to your training.

## CARDIO

Don't forget to put some cardio into your workout programme as well. By cardio, I mean some kind of physical activity that will raise your heartbeat like running or cycling. Cardio is good for your heart and entire cardiovascular system. It helps you burn energy and keeps the blood flowing. However, be careful not to do too much cardio and also avoid high intensity cardio. That would strip you of too much energy which you need for building your muscle fibres later on. The other problem is that high intensity cardio releases too many catabolic hormones into your body. If you want to do cardio, do low intensity cardio and keep your heart rate under 140 beats per minute. This level of cardio can help you with your recovery. By bringing some blood into your muscles, you clean waste products faster and bring your muscles the nutrients they need for recovery and growth. You will also provide them with more oxygen which again results in improved recovery. When you're trying to build some muscle, it's enough to include just 30-45 minutes of cardio in your programme once a week. Don't forget to calculate the energy expenditure and compensate for it in your diet. If you don't want to do cardio at all, you don't need to. Lot of people don't do cardio when they're building muscle and they get amazing results anyway. It's not something that determines your success.

However, it does speed up your recovery and keeps your cardiovascular system healthy. The latter is very important so if you don't want to do it regularly, do it at least once or twice a month. It's a pleasurable change for your body and it will help to keep your metabolism running properly.

# IX. Nutrition For Muscle Development

What you do outside the gym most influences your muscle growth. You'll spend around 4 hours a week in the gym and the rest of the time outside it. However, it's precisely that time outside the gym that determines whether you gain some muscle or not so make sure your rest and nutrition are of a high quality and quantity. The rules for your diet are simple. Make sure you receive enough protein and ensure you create a caloric surplus. Start with 2 grams of protein per 1 kilogram of your bodyweight, 5 to 9 grams of carbohydrates per 1 kilogram of your bodyweight and 0.5 to 1 gram of dietary fat per 1 kilogram of your bodyweight and then see how your body reacts to that. You can adjust it to your exact needs later on. However, don't forget about the variety in your diet as well. Besides macronutrients, you also need some vitamins and minerals so use this chapter to make sure your diet contains everything it's supposed to. The rules are very simple and if you follow them, your results will come relatively quickly. However, it's only up to you to follow them and that requires a certain amount of discipline.

**PROTEIN**

The first requirement of your muscle growth is sufficient protein intake. Protein is a basic building material for your muscle tissue. Its main use is recovery and building of new muscle fibres but it performs lot of other tasks as well. From the bodybuilding point of view, you only need to remember that the protein is a building material and your muscles fundamentally need it. You already know the answer to how much protein you need for your growth. It's 2 grams of protein per 1 kilogram of your bodyweight. Although you might see someone recommending eating 400 grams of protein a day in some magazines, this is completely misleading. You see, you can only build a certain muscle mass within a certain amount of time. It can sound like the more protein you eat, the more lean muscle tissue you can build. However, your hormone levels limit the amount of muscle you can build and so you don't need excessive amounts of protein. You can only use your hormone system as nature intended for you. If you receive more protein, your body won't use it for building more muscle anyway and if you receive less, it might not be enough for you. The smallest amount that still allows you to build muscle is 1.8 grams of protein per 1 kilogram of your bodyweight. As you get close to this limit, then muscle growth also depends on the rest of your food, especially carbohydrates. So, don't go below 1.8 grams of protein per 1 kilogram of your bodyweight. You might find it's not enough for building your muscle. And don't forget about getting enough carbohydrates and dietary fat along with your protein. Make sure you have sufficient amounts in your diet of each at all times so that there's nothing missing in your diet. Otherwise, you'll break down  the protein and use it for covering your total energy requirements instead of repairing and building your muscle tissue.

## ENERGY REQUIREMENTS

Your energy requirements during your body transformation will be mainly covered by your increased carbohydrate intake. The increased consumption allows you to create a caloric surplus that's needed for creating an anabolic environment. This anabolic environment will support your further muscle growth later on. Moreover, you will need extra energy for your workouts as well and this is why the importance of a caloric surplus is so crucial during your muscle development. But how do you know what level of caloric surplus you need? First of all, find out your basal metabolism and multiply it by the Physical Activity Factor. To do this calculation, you can use the Schofield Equation, which is described in the appendices at the end of this book. By using this calculation, you will find out how many calories you need for the maintenance of your current weight. Let's say you need around 2500 calories for maintaining your muscle. If you want to build some new muscle, you need to increase your daily caloric intake by at least 200 calories and receive 2700 calories a day. Your muscles will inevitably grow as a consequence. If that's not the case and you see no progress whatsoever, increase your daily caloric intake by another 200 or 300 calories. Your caloric intake will then equal 3000 calories a day and, even though you don't need to follow this number strictly, you at least need to know it so you get an idea of what to aim for. The number of carbohydrates needed along with those 2 grams of protein and 0.5 to 1 gram of fat per 1 kilogram of your bodyweight to create that caloric surplus is then calculated according to your daily caloric requirement.

## FOOD QUALITY

When you're choosing your meals, the most important factor is the food quality. Your muscles won't grow from pizza and chips or other foods with a low nutrient density. They will only grow if you receive the optimal amount of nutrients from the right kind of food. What you need is some protein, slow carbs, some natural sources of quick carbs and healthy fats and oils like nuts, olive oil or fish oils for example. If you eat lots of hamburgers, chips and cakes, you will only get fat and that has nothing to do with your body transformation at all. High quality food should make up at least 80% of your total food intake. If you want to have a cheat meal from time to time, feel free to have it. It will still help you to fulfil your caloric requirements. However, try to do without it. Sometimes you'll find yourself in a situation where you can't have the correct food you need and so you'll have to get a hamburger, sandwich or other fast food. Of course, you have to support your caloric intake in any way possible so make sure that this food is an exception and not a continuation of a series of unhealthy fast foods.

## A CHEAT DAY AND A CHEAT MEAL

Your food choices will start to narrow down during your body transformation. Chicken, fish, lean beef, eggs, rice, pasta, wholemeal pastry, nuts and vegetables and then again chicken, fish, lean beef, eggs, rice, pasta, wholemeal pastry, nuts and vegetables. Although they're high quality food, you will crave other food from time to time as well. Quick sugar, lots of fat and salt will call to you and the best thing to do is to plan for this kind of meal in advance. You might just want to plan one meal or you can even plan a whole day like this. A cheat meal is a meal where you don't care about your macronutrients and you only care about the taste of the meal. There are two kinds of people here: someone who eats these meals all day long and someone that just has one such meal once in a while. Which person you choose to be is up to you. If you want to have an entire cheat day, do it once every week. Eat two to three cheat meals during that day and something of nutritional value as well, of course. If you prefer only one cheat meal, have it every fourth or fifth day. You need to find for yourself the best option for you. One cheat meal in four days is not going to cause you to gain enormous amounts of fat and neither is one cheat day a week. However, be careful not to eat so much that you end up with an excess 2000 additional calories in your cheat meals. That would be a bit much!

## MEAL FREQUENCY

Try to eat regularly every two to three hours and eat at least 4 or 5 meals a day. This way, you will provide your body with consistent amounts of protein as well as the other nutrients you need. Although this kind of meal frequency is not necessary, it is optimal. If you're trying to put all your nutrients into three meals, your meals will be rather big and you will feel bloated after their consumption. However, if you split your daily intake into six meals, for example, you'll avoid this feeling and never get hungry. Everything depends on your preferences and also on your possibilities. If you prefer 5 meals a day, try eating 5 meals a day. If you prefer 5 meals a day Monday to Friday and 6 meals a day during the weekend, feel free to do whatever you prefer. At the end of the day, what matters most is the nutrient distribution in your diet so make sure you spread your nutrients across all of your daily meals. The important thing with your body transformation is to have enough protein and a caloric surplus. If you want to build some muscle, these two things have to be taken care of. Your nutrients can be received from 4 meals just as well as from 6 meals. It doesn't really matter that much. Those nutrients are being digested for longer then you rest between your meals anyway. Just make sure you don't eat less than 4 meals a day. It's partially about the speed of your digestive system but also about keeping your blood sugar levels stable throughout the day. If your days are very busy, alter the number of your meals accordingly so you can do everything you need during your day as well.

## MEAL TIMING

Getting your meal timing right can increase the effectiveness of your body's food utilization. It applies to two situations mainly: when you wake up in the morning and immediately after your workout. Your breakfast will help you start up your metabolism and top up the needed nutrients that you're missing. You see, your body can't access them during the night and that's why your body demands them in the morning. It'll also refill your energy stores, increase your blood sugar levels, top up the protein for your muscle building and get you set up for the rest of the day. This allows you to start your day very effectively. The other time when food is best used is after your workout, when your body is even more sensitive to food. Always eat something within the first hour after your workout. Your workout presents a huge exertion on your muscles and depletes your body of lots of energy. That means your body is crying out for food after your workout so it can suck all the nutrients out of it to use them. It needs to top up its depleted glycogen stores and repair the muscle tissue that you exercised during your workout. That's why you should really focus on getting food after your workout. Together with your breakfast, these two meals allow you to have some quick sugars too. Whilst complex carbohydrates are important, you need the energy as soon as possible in these two situations so feel free to have some quick sugars.

## APPETITE BOOST

When you switch to a higher food volume, you'll often find you don't have the appetite to eat everything that you're supposed to eat. This happens to a lot of people because they're used to lower food volumes and their metabolism is acting accordingly. They prepare the amount of food they're supposed to eat but struggle to eat it most of the time. They either feel full in the middle of the meal or they just skip the meal completely. So, if you find that happening and your appetite is low at the beginning of your muscle building adventure, you're not the only one who needs to solve this situation. You will need to overcome it like many others so stick to your nutritional plan for the first couple of days even though you don't have the appetite to sustain it. When you start feeling full during your meal, just carry on eating. You know how much food you need to eat in order to create a caloric surplus so eat it, even if you need to force yourself. You'll gradually pick up speed and the low appetite problem will vanish. The other group of people who might struggle at the beginning are the people who spend more than an hour at every meal. If you find you need to eat 5 meals a day and you spend an hour at each meal, your eating will take up practically your whole day and you won't want to eat your next meal because you've only just finished your last. Learn to eat a bit faster. You don't need to win a food eating competition but don't spend too much time with your food either. If you experience appetite loss in the later stages of your body transformation, take one or two days off from your dieting. Don't think about the contents or size of your food. Just eat when you're hungry and eat whatever you long for. You should regain your appetite very soon.

## MEAL PREPARATION

A really helpful and smart thing to do is to prepare several portions of food at once. Eat one portion immediately and save the rest for later. You'll cut your time spent in the kitchen and you'll always have some food ready. The worst thing that can happen to you when you're building muscle is when your meal is not ready and you don't have any food to use for something quick. Try to avoid these situations if possible because what you'll usually do in situations like this is go for pre-cooked meals with low nutrient density. That's not good for your metabolism and it increases the possibility of losing control and sliding into emotional eating. All of this can be simply avoided by preparing your meals in advance. It's the most convenient and easiest solution for you.

## RECIPE

Cooking doesn't have to be complicated. You don't need to cook healthy "fitness foods" described in various recipes. You don't have time for that. The important thing is for your meals to contain everything they should and for their preparation to be quick and easy. There are lot of other things on your agenda besides cooking and working out. If you want to cook by following recipes, you'll spend an enormous time on your cooking. A tasty meal can be prepared without any recipe whatsoever. You only need to know the nutritional value your meal is supposed to have and roughly how you're going to prepare it. If you've never cooked in your life, then do learn how to cook a bit. You will definitely need some cooking skills during your body transformation as you'll be preparing your meals almost every day. You don't need to cook at a five-star level because your muscle growth doesn't care about or grow according to how your meals taste. They only care about the nutrients therein. Nevertheless, you can make your meals a pleasurable experience for you. Season it to the best of your ability and enjoy it to the last bite. But still, don't waste your time by cooking complicated recipes you aren't familiar with.


## PERMANENT CHANGE


Your nutrition doesn't influence only your body but your mind as well. In other words, as you learn how to use your foods during your body transformation, you'll not only look better but you'll also think more clearly as your mental abilities improve as well. It would be nice if you carried on doing that for the rest of your life too. That might seem like part of the distant future right now but you will reach the time when you get to your goals and become satisfied with your physique. Promise yourself that when this time comes, you won't go back to your old eating habits again. Promise yourself that you'll stick to what helped you change your physique even after you reach your goals. If you're not interested in moving forward, at least maintain what you've got. You will feel better both physically and mentally. It's very easy to stop working on yourself and start enjoying your life too much again. The problem with this is that you may well end up back where you started so don't look at your body transformation as something that only lasts for a couple of weeks or months. Take care of your body for the rest of your life. The knowledge you'll gain and the experiences it brings will stop you from treating your body like a rubbish bin anyway. Once you get used to high-quality food, but then start eating something unhealthy and high in calories with lots of quick sugars and saturated fat, your body will immediately recognize it. Your concentration will drop, your mood will start swinging and you'll start putting on weight. Don't go back to your old eating habits because it's just not worth it; make sure that the change is for the long term.

## SUPPLEMENTS

The only supplements you need are whey protein and creatine as well as possibly multivitamins and fish oil. You don't need anything else. At some point, you'll meet someone who tells you that you need other supplements like glutamine, tribulus, beta-alanin and all kinds of other supplements. These substances might have some value but you don't need them. They're not bad in themselves but you'd waste your money because the two basic supplements mentioned above are sufficient for your muscle development. However, these can only help you if your nutrition is right, so make your diet your priority. Make sure your diet is as it's supposed to be and if you get it right, you will move forward whether you use supplements or not. Supplements merely provide speed for your progress. Eat high quality foods, use the mentioned supplements and work hard. If you do everything as you're supposed to, you will move forward and as long as you're moving forward, don't over-think it and stick to what's working.

**Part 4**
**Fat Loss**

# X.  Fat Loss Philosophy

If you want to lose fat, you have to change your eating and exercise habits. There are no short cuts so don't waste your time looking for them. Your body works according to some basic principles and neither your fat loss nor your muscle development are an exception to them. You have to learn why is fat stored in your body and the role of the nutrition and hormones in this process. If you discover the reason why your body stores excessive amounts of fat, you will be able to consciously eliminate it. Your fat storage will stop increasing and you will instead be able to work on decreasing it. Also, learn how to track your fat loss properly. Lots of people follow bodyweight measurements and these are very misleading. The following pages offer you an interesting insight on body fat storage and the measurement thereof.

## BODY FAT STORAGE

A healthy body needs some subcutaneous fat. It is part of a properly-functioning body and serves as an evolutionary backup, designed for when you can't get at food for some time. Therefore, fat is very beneficial and useful for your body. However, excessive fat storage is a problem. If you want to solve it, the first thing you need to do is to understand its origins. You need to understand that everything starts with your bad eating habits. If you eat too much food and your food choices are very poor, you will store fat as a consequence. Although food is your source of energy, you only need a certain amount of energy. Moreover, the energy received from your diet can only be utilised to a certain extent. If you receive more calories than your body needs, the excessive energy will start accumulating in your body as stored fat. It's a very simple mechanism that hasn't changed throughout history and it's not going to change any time soon. However, there is something else that needs to be said. Your total caloric intake and caloric expenditure are not the only cause of this problem because not all calories are made equal. The quality of your food, together with the source of your food, determines whether you become fat or not. That's why you also need to take a look at how the entire process of storing body fat is affected by your hormones. When it comes to hormones, you can alter them by making the right choices when it comes to food.

## DIET HIGH ON CARBOHYDRATES

Lot of fat people think they're fat because their diet is high in fat, which is not entirely true. Although bad nutritional fat plays a big part in damaging your health, it's not the sole reason for storing fat. The cause of storing excessive amounts of fat is something else. It is an excessive amount of carbohydrates. Carbohydrates affect your bodyweight more than any other macronutrient and are the main reason for getting fat.

The reason is that they cause a release of insulin. This stores fat in your fat cells, protein in your muscle cells and converts glucose into its storage form, glycogen. So, the more insulin there is in your blood, the more fat gets to your fat cells. If your body releases only small amounts of insulin, the fat is less able to get into the fat cells. Thus, the problem is in eating excessive amounts of carbohydrates. However, it's still a little more complicated. By eating huge amounts of carbohydrates, your body increases its resistance against insulin and various cells develop this resistance at a different pace. Liver cells create the resistance first, but fat cells take longer. So, when the liver cells develop the resistance against insulin but fat cells don't develop it yet, your liver releases lots of sugar into your bloodstream and the insulin sends a signal to your fat cells to store the fat that you receive from your foods. High insulin levels send a signal to your fat cells to store the fat and also increases their propensity for storing fat. As you eat carbohydrates, the insulin level in your bloodstream stays high and the fat that is supposed to feed all tissue in your body isn't released from your fat cells. Because your body can't access the fat stored in your fat cells, it gets hungry. The next thing you know, you're hungry and you decide to eat again. And the same thing happens again. Your body stores fat whilst being unable to access what it does have stored, thus getting hungry again. Eating too much carbohydrate becomes a vicious circle; your fat cells only get bigger and you simply get fatter.

## INSULIN AND GLUCAGON

Glucagon is, along with the insulin, equally important for your metabolic processes. Insulin and glucagon are the two hormones that affect the fat storage and fat release from your fat cells the most. Both hormones are released by your pancreas and both can be found in your blood at the same time. However, they perform the very opposite tasks. Insulin lowers the sugar levels in your blood, while glucagon raises them. Insulin sends your kidneys a signal to hold the water in your body, while glucagon sends them signal to get rid of it. Insulin stores the fat in your fat cells, while glucagon releases it from your fat cells. They are, essentially, opposites. The good news is that you can consciously affect their ratio in your blood. This can be done by monitoring your diet as various macronutrients cause various responses in your metabolism. Carbohydrates raise the amount of insulin in your blood but don't affect your glucagon levels. Protein slightly raises the level of both hormones whilst fat doesn't affect either that much. Thus, if you stick to getting protein from every meal, your insulin levels will stop sky-rocketing. This way, you'll minimize the fat storage and glucagon will become predominant. As a result, more fat will be released from your fat cells than is stored and you will gradually lose weight. So, if you decide to try a diet low in carbs, the glucagon dominance is what is going to bring you your desired success. However, don't forget that you still need to create a certain caloric deficit.

## CALORIE RESTRICTION

Every diet you ever heard of works on two principles only. The first principle is calorie restriction, which means you take less calories in than you need for maintaining your current bodyweight. The second principle is a correct ratio of macronutrients, referring again to the idea that all calories are not created equal. If you remember, this means that calories received in the form of protein are utilised in a different way in your body than the calories received from carbohydrates. That's why you can only lose fat if you change your eating habits. If you're trying to lose some fat for the first time, you will be fine with just eating 2 grams of protein per 1 kilogram of bodyweight and creating a caloric deficit. You will definitely manage to lose some fat. If you want to get to a really low body fat percentage, try the Cyclical Ketogenic Diet (CKD). It focuses on complete carbohydrate and insulin minimisation. This diet can do miracles for you if you do it right. However, you can get equally fantastic results from other numerous diets, based on those two principles that I mentioned above whether it's calorie restriction or specific macronutrient ratios.

## TWO TYPES OF FAT IN YOUR BODY

When it comes to fat loss, lot of people immediately think of the loss of their subcutaneous fat. However, subcutaneous fat is not the only type of fat in your body. Besides subcutaneous fat, there is visceral fat that is stored somewhere completely different. Subcutaneous fat is stored under your skin and is relatively harmless. However, if you have it in excess, your body looks rather fat. You can minimise it but you can't get rid of it entirely. The thing is that, you simply have to have some subcutaneous fat to function. Visceral fat, on the other hand, surrounds your inner organs. Excessive amounts of visceral fat cause the distance between your internal organs to increase and your waist looks wider. Moreover, you'll look like you have a beer belly. In general, men are more inclined to store this fat but women face the same issues after their menopause as well. If you weren't aware of visceral fat until now, that doesn't change your fat loss at all. You don't need to especially focus between the two types of fat right now. There aren't really any methods for that anyway. Just adjust your diet to reduce carbohydrates and calories a bit and then combine your lifting with some cardio. It's a simple solution that will help you minimize both types of fat at the same time.

## WEIGHT LOSS AND FAT LOSS

Another important thing to remember during your fat loss is that there is a difference between weight loss and fat loss. If you lose weight, it can be caused by burning fat and keeping muscle or by burning fat and muscle too. The ideal scenario is to achieve the first so that you burn some fat but keep your muscle. That is called fat loss. When you burn muscle along with your fat, you might be satisfied for a while. However, it's not an ideal solution from a long term point of view. You will miss the muscle you burn in the future. It's easy to lose muscle, but it's much harder to build it later. Thus, try to keep as much muscle mass as possible and only get rid of the fat. Fat loss can then lead to weight loss, although this isn't definite. If your body fat percentage is a little higher and you burn part of it, you will definitely lose some weight. However, if you're trying to decrease your body fat percentage by 2 or 3%, while you're relatively lean already, your bodyweight can easily stay where it is. Although you burn some fat, your bodyweight doesn't change. That is where a lot of people get confused. When they see no change in their bodyweight, they think nothing's happening. What they haven't realised is that their body composition has changed and that weight measurements don't explain this change. My point is that you shouldn't rely on your bodyweight as your sole indicator of progress during your body transformation. It won't provide you with a complete picture about how you're really doing.


## MEASURING BODY FAT


Measure your body fat percentage and body part circumferences as well. You can easily use a tape measure for measuring the circumference of your body parts. If you don't know how to measure your body fat, there are a couple of ways of doing it. The best thing to do is to use skin-fold callipers which can be easily bought online. You will be fine with just about any old skin fold callipers made of plastic. Usually, you also get a manual in the package explaining how to measure particular body parts and how to determine your overall body fat percentage based on your individual measurements too. However, if there's no manual, you can easily find the same information online. When you do measure with callipers, don't forget to allow for some margin of error when taking your measurements. Even skin-fold callipers won't give you a precise measurement all the time. However, it will give you a clear picture about your overall progress. Thus, skin fold callipers are a very good tool for you. If you use them during your body transformation, the measurements you get will give you absolute control over your progress.


## HEALTHY AND SUSTAINABLE LIMIT

The fastest progress during body transformation is experienced by the beginners. Their progress is fastest at its beginning and its speed depends on their starting point. For example, some beginners have a body fat percentage of about 30% and, therefore, huge room for improvement. It is much easier to get down to 15% body fat from 30% than to get from 10% down to 6% body fat. At 30% body fat, you can get fantastic results just by adjusting your diet and adding some training. Lot of people can get to a body fat percentage that is sustainable in the long run this way. In men, it's around 8 to 12% body fat and in women, it's around 20 to 25% body fat. So if you get to this level, be satisfied with yourself. This body fat percentage looks both healthy and aesthetic. However, lots of people are not satisfied even with this relatively low body fat percentage and try to get even lower. They either decide to test their limits or they want to get ready for a photoshoot. In these cases, men often aim for 6 to 7% body fat limit and women can get a similar definition at 13 to 14% body fat. If you want to do bodybuilding on a competitive level or you want to take a picture of your developed physique for whatever reason, you can try aiming for these levels. With the proper diet, training and discipline, it can be achieved relatively easily. You get to see your body well defined and it's an interesting experience. However, don't try to keep such a low body fat percentage for the long term. There's no reason for doing that. Not even professional bodybuilders keep low body fat percentages at all times. They only keep it for their competitive form. Permanently keeping body fat percentages this low can lead to hormonal problems.

## MORE MUSCLE EQUALS LESS FAT

The only way to solve the problem of body fat in the long term is to build some muscle. This overall muscle mass influences whether you store fat easily or not. Those aiming for weight-loss should be soothed by the fact that even 5  pounds of additional muscle encourage your body to burn more fat. However, when you spread these 5 lbs over your body, you won't be able to see that you've gained muscle. But, it really makes a difference to your energy-burning. A body that has a higher muscle mass burns more energy than a body that doesn't. That's why, if you lose a lot of weight and don't have enough muscle, it will be hard for you to keep that body fat percentage low. You will either go back to your normal diet and start gaining your weight back or you will have to control your diet and keep your daily energy intake down. But, if you try to maintain your weight by always having to stay away from something, it's not much of an achievement either. In the long term, the most convenient way of losing fat is building more muscle. More muscle means higher energy requirements for your body and gives you the opportunity to stay lean without having to control your diet all the time. However, having less control of your diet doesn't mean you can start eating hamburgers, chips and pizza every day. You still mainly need to stick to quality food. The advantage is that you don't have to control the amount of your food that much.

## TRANSFORMATION ROCKET APPLICATION

As this chapter closes, let's have a look at how to apply the Transformation Rocket to your fat loss.

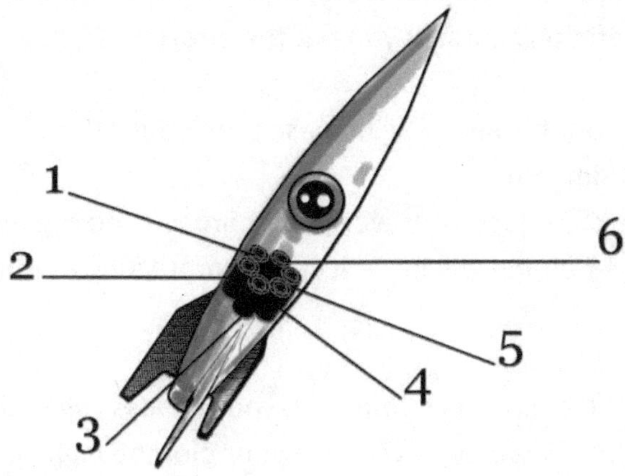

*1. Decision 2. Discipline 3.Time 4. Training 5. Nutrition 6. Supplementation*

1. Decision – Fat loss is psychologically more demanding than muscle building. The reason for this is that you have to create a caloric deficit during your fat loss and that can be reflected in your mood. That's why you need to decide in advance that a bad mood will not discourage you from continuing with your fat loss before you see the results you want. Decide to give your fat loss as much time and energy as is needed.

2. Discipline – You often won't feel like getting up and doing some running either. However, you know why you're doing that so keep your reason at the forefront of your mind. You always need to be disciplined. This doesn't just apply to your training only but to your nutrition as well. Pay attention to your daily caloric intake and don't eat inappropriate foods.

3. Time – If you want to change something about your body, it's not going happen overnight. The optimal sustainable speed of burning fat is 1 to 2 pounds of fat a week so (depending on your goals) you need to work at this for some time. The minimum time needed to notice a small

change is about three weeks so be prepared to test your patience. Your results will definitely come if you put the effort in.

4. Training – Your training will increase both your caloric expenditure as well as burn some fat.
You'll be able to choose your workout approach and the effort put into the resistance training will be reflected in protecting as much muscle as possible.

5. Nutrition – If you neglect your diet, your fat loss will end up right where it begins. However, if you give your diet the highest priority, your progress will not only surprise everyone around you but it will surprise you too. Just make sure you create a caloric deficit every day and your body will have to go into your fat storage to get some more energy.

6. Supplementation – If you're preparing for fat loss, you might think you don't need any supplements. However, remember that even during your fat loss, you're still working with your muscles and your job is to protect your muscle tissue as much as possible. Muscle mass is key to maintaining a low body fat percentage in the long run. Again, it's in your best interest to buy at least whey protein and creatine.

# XI.  Fat Loss Workout Structure

Similarly to your muscle development, your fat loss workouts will take place in the gym. Weightlifting is very important for the maintenance of your muscle so don't rely solely on your cardio. Although it can help you to burn some energy, it's not that effective for your muscle protection and your physique development. Moreover, the majority of aerobic activities put an asymmetrical load on your body. For instance, with cycling, your legs, bottom and back are worked far harder than your chest or arms. Running and other activities are very similar so if you only do cardio to lose weight, your body aesthetics will remain neglected. As one of the reasons for losing some fat is to look your best, make lifting the basis of your fat loss plan. It will allow you to target all your muscle groups equally, encouraging a good aesthetic. Moreover, you send your muscles a signal to remain strong and to remain equally big. The only way how to achieve this is by lifting heavy. Lot of people try to lose fat by converting lifting into cardio. They decrease their weights and increase the number of reps instead. However, they start losing their muscle mass because they don't need big muscles for lifting relatively light weights. The way to avoid this and to maintain as much muscle tissue as possible is to keep up with your resistance training and to always lift heavy.


## FULLBODY WORKOUT AND WORKOUT SPLIT


Whether you choose to do a fullbody workout or a workout split is again completely up to you. Both approaches fit their purpose equally well. Your choice purely depends on your preference. Some people like workout splits and some like fullbody workouts. People from both camps achieve amazing results so choose whatever suits you best and then stick to it. The only difference worth mentioning is that a fullbody workout will help you burn more energy. However, that's irrelevant since resistance training isn't part of your plan for energy burning but for your muscle and strength maintenance. So, don't make a decision between fullbody workout and workout split based on their caloric expenditure potential. Calorie burning will be covered by the cardio in your plan. If your diet and cardio help you create the caloric deficit, you'll keep losing weight regardless of whether you do fullbody workouts or a workout split in the gym. Instead, just make your decision based on what suits you the most.

## COMPOUND EXERCISES

The base of your workout will again be compound exercises. They were the base for your muscle development and they are the base of your fat loss as well. There's no reason to change those exercises whatsoever. Compound exercises are the most effective and most rewarding. With every exercise, more muscle groups are engaged which allows you to lift relatively heavy. That means a bigger load on your system over all. Only two things will change compared to the factors that relate to your muscle development; your workout intensity and your workout volume. You will do less sets in the gym and your rest interval will be longer. As a result, you will put less load on your body over all. However, because of the decreased workout intensity, make sure you use compound exercises only. The thing is that you need to put the most effort into those compound movements so if you want to add some isolated movements into your workout, add just one or two exercises maximum. Compound movements are far more effective than isolated ones when it comes to fat loss.

## HEAVY WEIGHTS

Similarly to your muscle development, you should lift heavy during your fat loss. The fact that you decrease your caloric intake and add some cardio into your training doesn't mean you need to change anything about your resistance training. You still need to keep as much muscle mass and strength as possible. One day, when you get to a body fat percentage level that will allow you to see your muscles clearly, you will finally be able to appreciate the aesthetics of your body. Lifting heavy will ensure your muscles look hard and developed so don't decrease your weight and don't change your rep range. Keep doing 6 to 12 reps and always try lifting heavy. If you're afraid you'll run out of energy, don't. Lowering the workout intensity and volume will ensure that you'll be able to handle it. Your rest interval between sets will be 2 to 3 minutes and your workout volume will decrease by one third which means that you will do less sets in your workouts. Remember that it's not about building muscle mass but about maintaining as much as you can during your fat loss. Although you can't stay away from some muscle loss, you can most certainly minimize it. That's why your workout intensity and workout volume will decrease and the number of days in a gym might decrease as well. It depends on how your muscles are responding to your training. It's better to have a proper workout with heavy weights and get one additional day of rest then to be easy on yourself, lower your weights and leave yourself some margins.

## REST INTERVAL

One of the things that will change compared to building muscle is your rest interval. Longer rests between your sets will give you enough time for both recovery and preparation for another set. This is important because you will get tired more easily during your fat loss. Your glycogen stores will almost always be empty and you'll be able to feel it. That's why your rest between sets will increase to about 2 minutes. Less than 2 minutes probably won't be enough for your muscles to recover while you're working with a lower energy intake so let them rest for longer. The indicator of success is your ability to get into that 6 to 12 rep range in your next set again. The length of your workout won't be affected either. Although your rest interval will be longer, you will do less sets. Your workout intensity won't be as high and the length of your workout will stay at around 45 to 60 minutes. If you can't keep up with this rest interval, you either need a longer rest or you picked a weight that's too heavy for you.

## REP RANGE

Your rep range stays at 6 to 12 again so there's nothing different here compared to plans for muscle development. Lots of people decrease their weight and increase the number of reps during their fat loss. They go up to 12 to 20 reps and think that's standard for fat-burning. They forget about protecting their muscle fibres and make their lifting into cardio. However, there is no such a thing as a 'rep range for fat loss'. If you change your rep range like this, you'll have problems maintaining your muscle tissue and your metabolic rate will drop as a consequence which is not a good thing. If you want to lose fat, adjust your caloric intake and start doing some cardio but don't change the structure of your workouts, your rep range or the weight of your resistance. If you start losing strength during your fat loss, adjust your weights so you can work in the same rep range again. Remember to always adapt your training to your current performance so it's challenging for you, always strive to lift more and always make sure you stay in that rep range of 6-12.

## ADAPTABILITY TO STRESS

Do some cardio along with your resistance training. Its purpose is to increase your energy expenditure and to support more fat burning. Technically, your fat loss can be done without doing the cardio at all. However, your diet needs to be exceptional for that and you need to lift weights to burn fat. However, if you're not trying to get to military-like conditions, just let it go. Keep a balanced diet and add some cardio to your workout programme. When you add the energy burned during your cardio to your daily expenditure, you will be able to raise your energy intake. You only need to stay 200 to 300 calories under your basic weight-maintaining needs and by doing this, you will be burning fat with a smile on your face. However, be aware of one very important shortcoming only known by a handful of people. Your body adapts to your cardio and so your cardio starts to lose its effectiveness over time. If you constantly want to burn the same amount of energy with your cardio, you either need to run faster or you need to run longer. However, if you increase your speed or the length of your cardio too much, the effectiveness of your cardio will start decreasing.

## CARDIO INTENSITY

During your cardio, your heart should be beating at 120 to 140 heartbeats per minute. That basically means that you should be able to keep a conversation during your cardio. If you're not able to keep a conversation going during your cardio, you're working too hard and your heartbeat is probably too high. Focus on your workout and on your breathing. Maintain your intensity and avoid increasing it. But don't focus too much on stretching your stamina limits because after all, you're not trying to win a 1500 meter run. When you do too much cardio, your body starts taking energy not only from your fat but from your muscles as well and this is not the aim. This is why you need to make sure you keep your heartbeat at around 120 to 140 beats per minute during your cardio. More than this and you'll miss your goal of a long-term body transformation.


## RESISTANCE TRAINING AND CARDIO RATIO

You might be wondering what ratio of cardio and resistance training is the best. The answer is really simple. Engage with them equally. Start with an equal amount of time and adjust it if you think you need to. The time spent on your resistance training is calculated depending on your workout programme, and the time you spend on cardio should match the former. Although the rough idea is that you spend equal times on cardio and resistance, the amount of cardio needed during a fat loss is individual. For example, try splitting it like this. Spend 45 minutes lifting weights in a gym and when you finish that, go for 15 minutes of cardio. On your non-lifting days, do 30 or 45 minutes of cardio. Don't overthink this ratio between resistance training and cardio too much though. It's not going to determine whether you lose some fat or not. Fat loss is mainly determined by your total energy intake and expenditure.

## WHEN TO DO YOUR CARDIO

The best time to do your cardio is right after your resistance training. The reason for doing resistance training and cardio in this order is obvious. By doing resistance training first, you work your muscles and use up your stored glycogen. So, when you do your cardio after your resistance training, your body will go straight into your fat storage for energy. The type of the cardio you do is completely up to you. You can choose any cardio machine and feel free to swap them every now and then. One day, use a bike and the next time, use something else. In order to avoid boredom, feel free to swap your cardio regularly. It also stops your body from getting used to the activity which would make your cardio start losing its effectiveness.  After 3 weeks of running, try cycling for the next 2 weeks. After that, you can try swimming or something else. It's up to you. There aren't any formulae for this. Just follow your intuition. A change will always help and if you don't want to change the actual activity itself, change the environment in which you do it. Swap between running indoors and outdoors. Although it's the same activity for your body, your mind will perceive it as a change. You will be more enthusiastic about your workout and you will avoid the plateau as well. The only thing you need to be careful about is not to change the surface types you do your cardio on too often. Getting used to those different surface types all the time would mean an excessive load for your joints, ligaments and tendons.

## FUN WITH YOUR CARDIO

There are lots of opportunities for cardio on your non-lifting days. The best thing you can do is to do your cardio somewhere outside on the fresh air. Both your health and your psyche will benefit from it. Sit on your bike or put your trainers on and indulge yourself in 45 minutes of cycling or running at a low intensity. If you don't enjoy these, do something else. Include some seasonal sports. During the summer, go swimming or play some tennis. If you're a fan of team sports, play football or basketball. During the winter, go skiing, snowboarding or play some ice hockey. Cardio doesn't have to be boring. You don't have to run the same route all the time and get bored. Call your friends and play some sports. Cardio will become both fun and a workout at the same time. Although you won't be measuring distance or keeping a proper heartbeat frequency, that's not especially important here. You will burn energy, spend some time with your friends and have a great time. Sometimes this is more important than measuring the exact numbers.

## DAY OFF

Don't forget to take at least one day off during your week. There will be more than enough workload during your fat loss and exhaustion will come as a consequence. Therefore, you need to relax every now and then. Your workouts will be hard and, if you want to train without rest, sooner or later there will be a price to pay. Sometimes, less is more and it pays to relax. If you're afraid that your day off is a breach of your discipline and you don't move forward that day, don't be. One day off during a week will give you so much more than working out again. You'll allow your muscles to recover and you'll get some rest. You won't end up with a big caloric surplus. Resistance training will enforce a higher energy expenditure the day after (which might be your day off). A day off is also prevention against injury. If you're trying to push your limits and your diet is low on calories, the exhaustion will start to accumulate and the risk of injury will creep into your workouts. Injury is the last thing you want during your body transformation.

## RECOVERY AND REST

Recovery and rest are very important parts of your body

transformation. The reason I am stressing this is because lots of people tend to neglect their recovery. However, your body needs recovery and not just to avoid injury. It's also for repairing and building new muscle fibres. Your body needs to top up your exhausted glycogen stores, it needs proper sleep and it sometimes needs an afternoon nap as well. Give yourself a couple of days when you do literally nothing of a physical nature. Without recovery, you won't get results. If you want to build muscle, you need to give your body time to actually do so. Your muscles don't grow in the gym; they grow when you get some nice rest and proper food after your workout. With your fat loss, it's exactly the same. If you train too much, you don't only burn your fat but your muscles too. Less muscle means a slower basal metabolism and a higher chance that you will gain that fat back again in the future. If you've got caught in the quick-lifestyle trap then it's highly likely you don't rest that much during the day. However, find some time for the rest during your day. You will definitely need it during your body transformation because your body and your results depend on it.

# XII. Nutrition For Fat Loss

Changing something overnight is extremely difficult and your diet is no exception to this. If you don't usually care about what and how much you eat, you won't change it overnight. Trying to change something overnight is a recipe for failure. Moreover, if you fail at this unrealistic goal, you will also gain painful memories which will later cause you to avoid trying it again. Introduce the change gradually instead. Find out how you need to change your diet and change it step-by-step. After time, you will develop some new habits and a new eating regimen. The time it takes depends only on you and your determination. However, decide on the speed you feel comfortable with and don't rush. Gradual change is the key to permanent change.

## WHAT TO EAT FOR FAT LOSS?

Start with creating a caloric deficit. Your daily caloric intake should be around 300 to 500 calories lower than you need for maintaining your current bodyweight. Gradually decrease the amount of carbohydrates in your diet and replace them with protein and fats. This way, you will start getting closer to a low carb diet even though you'll stay at the same amount of calories. The only thing that will change will be the amount of your macronutrients. The choice of foods will remain roughly the same as with muscle gain; mainly chicken, turkey, lean beef, fish, eggs, oats, sweet potatoes, brown rice, vegetable, nuts, seeds, different types of oils and so on. However, when it comes to carbohydrates, eat mainly slow carbs. This way, you can avoid a release of excessive insulin. Moreover, the fats received from your food will be used directly as a source of energy. So, you really need to make sure that there is a sufficient amount of fat in your diet. It might be strange to have sausage, steak and eggs on your plate when you're trying to burn fat but it really works. If you don't believe it, just try it and you'll see it yourself.

## PROTEIN IN EVERY MEAL

It's also important that every meal you eat should contain some protein. Protein is not digested that easily and some of the calories you receive from your food are used for digestion. This is called the thermic effect of food and it can only help you to get your results during your fat loss. However, these benefits are not the only advantage that you get from eating protein. It also prevents your blood sugar levels from rising too high. That would mean a release of excessive amount of insulin again and that is something you ideally want to avoid. Moreover, the protein will leave you with a good feeling of fullness so you won't feel hungry as fast as when you eat only carbohydrates.

Besides, don't forget that the protein in every meal provides you with enough building material for your muscles and muscle fibres. Keeping as much muscle as possible is very important. So the ideal scenario is to eat 5 to 6 meals a day and each of them containing some protein.


## IT'S ABOUT INSULIN


Be careful about eating quick carbs. During your fat loss, it will be very important how you can watch your insulin levels raised by quick carb consumption. Insulin's job is to consequently lower that high sugar in your blood again so if you eat a meal that contains carbohydrates, make sure those carbohydrates are slow carbohydrates. Instead of white rice, eat brown rice or sweet potatoes. The energy you will get from them will be released slowly and gradually. Limit your quick carbs intake to your breakfast and post-workout meal. It's in these two moments that a 'glycogen window' opens for you and it allows you to process the nutrients more effectively. Quick carbs are safe at these two moments. If you have no idea as to which carbohydrates are quick and which are slow, their glycaemic index will reveal it to you.
A glycaemic index shows how quickly sugar is released from foods into your body. The quickest carbohydrate is glucose with a glycaemic index of 100 and the lower the GI number, the slower the food's sugar is released into your bloodstream. Glycaemic index tables can be found anywhere online. They'll give you an overview as to which foods are desirable.


## LEMON AND LIME


One of the tricks of decreasing the sugar levels in your blood and insulin in your body is the consumption of soluble fibre. Fibre helps with the movement of the food in your digestive system and bonds with cholesterol. It can be divided to soluble fibre and insoluble fibre. Soluble fibre absorbs large amounts of water while, by contrast, insoluble fibre doesn't absorb any water. Insoluble fibre can be found mainly in wheat products, vegetables and fruit; soluble fibre can be found in barley and oat products and seeds. The best source of soluble fibre are pears and citrus fruits. A distinctive advantage that soluble fibre has is that they help you to lower your blood sugar levels which means less released insulin overall. Sugar from your foods will be absorbed more slowly into your body and you will feel full for longer. Let's go back to the fact that soluble fibre can be found in citrus fruits. When you're on a fat loss, lemons and limes are an amazing combination. From these two, you can receive the soluble fibre while they contain minimum amounts of carbohydrates. The best thing you can do when you're going to eat lots of quick carbs is to drink a big glass of water with lemon or lime juice before your meal. That will help you slower your insulin response. Also, besides the juice, try to find a way to ingest the pith and peel of these fruits. There is far more soluble fibre in the skin than there is in any other part of these fruits. However, drink no more than 2 or 3 glasses of this mixture per day. Lemon and lime can have side effects in large amounts as well.

## AVOID EATING TOXIC THINGS

Avoid both white and brown sugar. Both types of sugar are so bad for your body. They cause a very high insulin response which leads to all kinds of problems, whether you're into fitness or not. In the long term, they destroy your teeth, heart and digestive system. Sugar is the cause of diabetes type II, cardiovascular problems, high levels of bad LDL cholesterol and high blood pressure. Nevertheless, people eat it because of its unbelievably delicious taste. Its sweet taste stimulates a part of your brain that releases a substance called dopamine into your body as a reward. This means that when you eat some sugar, there is a response in your body similar to the one you get with alcohol or drugs like cocaine. That's the reason why people have always desired sugar and always will. White sugar, brown sugar, syrups, sweet foods and soft drinks all mean damage to your body. So, if you love your body, stay away from the refined sugar. Eating sugar is similar to misfueling your car. If you use some gimmicky 'super-fuel' rather than petrol, you'll have problems so be careful about the sugar consumption. You can't avoid it completely because it already is in your diet. However, avoid unreasonable consumption. It's similar to alcohol and tobacco which are both toxic substances for your body. If you get your sugar from fruit, you will get all the fibre, minerals, protein, fats and enzymes as well. This is okay and your body can cope with that blend of substances. However, digesting refined sugar is quite the digestive battle and detracts from your overall level of health so stay away from it.

## DIETARY FAT

Dietary fat is often mentally linked with flabby bellies, thighs and bottoms so most people think it's bad. However, weight gain is not caused by dietary fat consumption. On the contrary, dietary fat is very important for your body and your body utilizes it in various, necessary ways. Nevertheless, be careful about the type of fat you consume. Monosaturated fats, polyunsaturated fats and omega-3 fatty acids are 'good fats', things your body needs. They can be found in olive oil, aubergines, peanut butter, nuts and soy. Make sure you get enough of them staying under your established daily energy intake at the same time. On the other hand, be careful about saturated fats and transfatty acids. They can be found in chicken skin, margarine, butter and other foods. They help to raise the level of your bad cholesterol and equally raise the risk of cardiovascular diseases. Ideally, you'll avoid them. You need to differentiate between the fats that you include in your diet because not all fats are equal. Some are detrimental to you and some are beneficial. Focus on eating enough of those beneficial and minimize the presence of those detrimental. Those beneficial fats are not the reason you're overweight and you must make sure you get enough of them.

## A CHEAT DAY AND A CHEAT MEAL

If you want to have a high calorie meal, plan it in advance. Don't get seduced by these meals every time you get some cravings. Resist. Additional calories can spoil all your hard work very easily. At the beginning, it all seems very innocent and you think that you'll only take a small portion. However, high calorie meals are delicious and before you notice it, a small portion turns into a big one. Instead of giving in, try holding back for a couple of days and then reward yourself with a cheat day or a cheat meal. Do it as a part of your plan. Plan for one cheat day every week and eat, for example, 3 cheat meals during such a day. However, don't think you need to eat tons. Cheat days aren't for feeding up but for satisfying your taste and doing the least harm possible to your body. It also serves to introduce something new to your metabolism. Just like cardio, your metabolism gets used to your diet after some time and a cheat day keeps it on its toes. However, a cheat day will cause your bodyweight to rise the next day. The majority of this weight will be only water and refilled glycogen stores so, if you've lost some weight during a week and you gain about 0.5 kilograms after a cheat day, it's not a matter of gaining 0.5 kilograms of fat during that day and there's no need to feel sad or worried. It's only water and glycogen stores. However, if you can't lose fat in the long term, limit your cheat day to only one cheat meal a week.

## MEAL FREQUENCY

Keeping regular breaks between meals is not that important. Whether you lose some weight or not is determined by a caloric deficit and a ratio of macronutrients in your diet and not by your eating routine. Just look at the people that achieve great results with intermittent fasting. Their daily nutrition intake is compressed into 4- to 8-hour windows whilst eating nothing during the rest of the day and they still achieve amazing results. Nevertheless, I still recommend eating approximately every 3 hours. It will help you to control your hunger. If your break between two meals is 5 or 6 hours, you're far more likely to get hungry and end up eating cake or chips. Regular breaks between meals ensure that you feel full throughout the day. However, if you aren't able to do this, it's not a problem. Instead, plan your meals so they're convenient for you.

## WORKING OUT ON AN EMPTY STOMACH

Never skip your breakfast. Lots of people think it's better to train with an empty stomach and so they skip their breakfast. They think that, if they train with an empty stomach, it will help them burn more energy. However, it's not like that. If you don't eat before your morning workout, you simply put your muscle fibres in danger. Your body will start looking for the energy everywhere and it will start getting it from your muscle tissue. You want to keep as much muscle as possible and therefore you ideally want to avoid this scenario. Start your morning with breakfast. It will give you the energy you need in order to push your limits during your workout. Without breakfast, you'll feel weak and that will limit your performance so don't skip your breakfast. What's going to matter the most at the end of the day is the caloric deficit that you will create. If you know that you're going to meet this requirement, there is no reason to skip your breakfast and deplete yourself of the energy needed for your workout.

## LACK OF ENERGY DURING YOUR WORK

When you start creating a caloric deficit, your energy levels may fall. If you have a manual job, you will notice it immediately and your muscles will let you know about it straight away. However, if you have a non-manual job, it will show up as a loss of concentration and an overall exhaustion. Your brain requires some energy for working properly and a lack of easily-available energy can have a negative influence on your mental work. Long-term poor performance and a bad temper are two signs that something's wrong. If you feel exhausted for long periods of time and you lose your concentration often, your caloric deficit is probably too big. So if you're trying to eat 1000 calories less a day, alter this to 500 calories less a day. The thing is that, no matter how much you want to lose weight, you need to avoid absolute exhaustion. From a long term point of view, a caloric deficit of about 500 calories a day is better. Of course, if you embark on a low carb diet, where the majority of foods consists of protein and fat, the problem is somewhere completely different. Low energy levels during low carb diets are related to a lack of dietary fats in your diet or a lack of water needed for your metabolism. So if you feel tired, add more fats into your diet. In this scenario, your body needs them as a source of energy.

## SALT AND WATER

If adding more dietary fat doesn't help and you start experiencing dizziness and weakness, something's wrong. The truth is that lot of people experience this during a low carb diet. It occurs mainly at the beginning of the new dietary regimen, when their body starts reacting to a limited carbohydrate intake. Your kidneys start removing the stored water and what leaves your body along with the water are salts. A lack of salts consequently causes your body to flush incoming water and you get dehydrated. People don't know this can happen during a low carb diet and they don't prepare for that. Next thing you know, they feel weakness, exhaustion, dizziness, headaches and low mental alertness. That's why you need to watch your daily water intake carefully so you don't get dehydrated. Exhaustion without these other signs might be caused by the lack of energy, but if you experience dizziness, headaches and similar signs together, you definitely need more water and more salts. Start putting more salt into your meals and if that doesn't help, get some supplements containing potassium.

## HUNGER AND CRAVINGS

Another consequence of your diet adjustment will be hunger. If you decrease the amount of carbohydrates and the total amount of food in your diet, you will be hungry from time to time. Your body will tell you it needs food in order to survive. Hunger in itself is good because it serves to keep you out of danger. However, you're not going to starve as long as you have healthy eating habits during your fat loss and if you get hungry anyway, drink a glass of water. Hunger is often just a reflection of thirst and having a drink should remove the feeling of hunger. If you're still hungry, you'll just need to grin and bear it. Fat loss is sometimes about self-control as well. One solution can be keeping 3 to 4 hour breaks between your meals. This way, you will easily be able to cope until you have another meal. At the beginning, you might experience some hunger and cravings for something sweet or unhealthy but, as you get used to it, you will get used to your new eating regimen.

## SMALLER PLATES

Adjustments in your diet will also cause the volume of your daily food intake to shrink. There are things you can do so this doesn't affect you psychologically. Here's a really easy way. Use smaller plates. This is a great trick for putting less food on the plates and still keeping the feeling that your plate is full. It leaves you with a visual feeling of plentitude and abundance. It's just a small trick but it can help you in a big way. If you don't want to use smaller plates, fill your plate with some salad. Something low in calories that is beneficial in your diet at the same time. Again, you will get the impression that your plate is full. Just be creative and look for ways to avoid situations when you think you're fed up with your fat loss. Look for ways to make a pleasurable activity out of your fat loss, to enhance your results and to keep yourself psychologically relaxed at the same time.

# Part 5

# The Approach

## XIII. What to expect

The hardest part that comes with every change is the beginning. Anything you do requires conscious thought and everything will be relatively new for you. Certainty and confidence are only built over time. Remember that all these events wait for you during your body transformation too. The first week might be very hard. You'll start going to a gym, you'll change your diet and start taking some supplements too. Your workouts will take all of your energy and you will feel tired. It will be very hard on you, both physically and psychologically. However, although the first days will be very difficult, you'll get used to it very soon. You'll get used to your new daily routine and you'll start doing lot of things automatically. You'll get used to your journey to the gym, to your supplements and your body will get used to the stress in the gym. Once you pass these early stages, the rest of the time will be much easier on you.

## YOUR ENERGY LEVELS

Your energy levels will change during your first week too. How they'll change depends on whether you need to lose fat or gain muscle. If you need to lose some fat, you need to take in less calories than you are used to. Therefore, you will lack some energy during your first week. You will notice it during physical work as well as during mental work. Your body will struggle for a couple of initial days and you will be tired. But, after a couple of days, you'll get used to it and even though your tiredness won't disappear completely, it won't cause you any problems either. It works the same when you're building some muscle. The only difference is that your caloric intake will be higher and you will have more energy. This energy will have to be expressed somehow so if your mood goes up and down in extremes, don't be surprised. Everything happens for a reason and, in this case, the reason is just that you have extra energy.

## YOUR LIFESTYLE

As I've said, a lot of things are going to change at the beginning of your journey. Body transformation won't just be a challenge for you, it will become your lifestyle. Developing your body isn't like other sports or hobbies. If you want to be successful, you need to give it everything you've got. Body transformation is a matter of non-stop effort towards changing every little thing that affects your body. It's not enough to do things right once and it's not enough to do them right every now and then. You need to do them right all the time. It is a lifestyle. If you're willing to do everything as needed, your body will willingly shape according to your vision. It's only about you and what you want. You can't do this kind of thing half-heartedly. You need to put yourself into it with all your body, mind and soul. Lot of people don't understand that they simply won't get results otherwise. Sometime they have a workout and sometimes not. Sometimes they have a chicken salad for a lunch and sometimes they have a big hamburger with chips. This is not the way it works. Body transformation requires a non-stop approach. Your lifestyle needs to be in line with your goals.

## USE YOUR WILLPOWER

So, decide to give your body transformation everything you've got. It will help you get through the hard times which you will certainly encounter. This commitment to fully immerse yourself in your body transformation will become critical. Let's say you're trying to build some muscle. However, instead of growth, you will experience a plateau and don't make any progress for a few days. A few days will roll into a few weeks and you'll become nervous. Your training is perfect, your nutrition is perfect but there's no progress. What will you do? Will you give up or will you use your willpower and give it everything you've got? Your willpower will help you push harder to move forward. It's one of the keys to success. Pain on your last reps, exhaustion on your last kilometre and other demanding situations will require your will to be strong. If you have a strong will, you're one step ahead. If you have a strong will, you will make a difference, even in those tiniest details. You will complete that last rep when you feel you can't go on and you will lift that slightly heavier weight even though it hurts.

## EXERTION BOUNDARY

However, be careful to know what's reasonable and what's not. You're not in this to torture your body. If you go to the gym twice a day, 7 days a week, you won't have any time for recovery which you'll sorely need. You need to top up your energy stores and allow your muscle fibres to recover. If you train too often, you will simply overtrain yourself. Eventually, it can discourage you and you might decide to quit your body transformation. Rather than this dire situation, choose a smarter way and don't try to be a hero. At the end of the day, you're the only one losing out. With such an enormous exertion, you're exposed to various injuries. Your body is tired and its immunity decreases. Think about where the exertion boundary and the point at which your effort just doesn't make any sense any more might be.

## PATIENCE

Everybody wants everything instantly. Nobody has any spare time and everyone seems to be too busy. If you order food, you want it immediately. If you buy something online, you want it delivered straight away. You need it right now because next week is going to be too late already! Pressure from all around us has taught us to expect things instantly. However, there is a small problem with this attitude. You can't actually have everything immediately. Do you want to get rich? It's not going to happen overnight. You need a proven plan that you'll be working on very hard. Do you want to learn a new language? That's not going to happen overnight either. Even the cleverest of people need a couple of months to do it. Do you want to transform your body? That will take some time too. You need to work on it for a while because it's a process like everything else. You can maximize its speed but you can't make a giant leap within a couple of hours or days. Body transformation requires some patience on your part.

## DISCIPLINE

It also requires some discipline. You have a goal, you have a winning plan and you're hungry for success. Add discipline and you will get your results very soon. Train one hundred percent, eat what your body needs and make sure your food has the necessary nutritional value. No hamburgers, no crisps, no cakes. Get decent sleep during the night and don't waste your energy in clubs. There is no such thing as a nightlife when transforming your body. When the weather is cold outside, wear a jacket and care about your health. A body that's not healthy can't make any progress. No alcohol. No drugs. You have a goal so work on it. And you made yourself a promise, so live up to it. Disciplined people always achieve their goals. They know what they want and they go after it. Disorderly people either don't know what they want or they don't want it enough. You can be one of these two people; either you have discipline or you don't. If you don't already have discipline, start work on it now. Sport is the perfect activity for acquiring it and body transformation twice so.

## PAIN

That last rep in a gym, that last kilometre of your run or even the thought of one of these will give you some pain at times. They won't only hurt during your actual exercise but after the exercise or when the thought of exercising crosses your mind can be painful. But that's okay! Pain is exactly what helps you to move forward so don't see it as something bad. You can't get to your new body without some pain. It's just left-overs from your previous weakness. Pain will stop eventually but what comes after is pure strength. Think of working through pain as a sign of your progress. Every time you feel pain, you have only two options. You either give up and the pain will go away or you sustain it and give it your best, eventually overcoming it properly. Choosing the latter is right when you start moving forward. It is at that moment that you give your body a signal to adapt to your new requirements. It is right then that you form your personality. When you learn how to work with pain and you start utilizing it for your development, you stop worrying about it and you will even start searching for it because without pain, there is no progress at all. If your training doesn't challenge you, it doesn't change you.

## ATTITUDE

Everything depends on your attitude. A sloppy attitude leads to sloppy results. The right attitude leads directly to your goals. It's a small detail that makes a big difference in your life. That's why it's important to have the right attitude towards your body transformation. You should always feel good about it because lots of different things are going to happen. There will be good, funny and valuable things but also bad, unpleasant and difficult things. How you cope with them depends mainly on your attitude. The better your attitude is, the better you can deal with them. If you couldn't complete the number of reps that you planned in one set on your squats today, what are you going to do about it? Are you going to be sad and mope around? Are you going to blame everyone around you because you couldn't focus? Will you get angry? Nothing like that will help you. Find a way to complete the reps next time and consider it a challenge instead. Stay calm and get that number of reps next time. Go to bed 30 minutes earlier, watch your diet more closely, play your favourite music and you will make it.

# XIV. Commitment, fulfilment and joy

Only you can change your body and nobody else can do it for you. This is why it's so important to know exactly what you're doing. Learn the basic principles of training and nutrition and find out how to use them. Join your gym and get used to the environment in which you'll be working on yourself. Learn how to breath and exercise properly. Notice how your body reacts to your workouts. Learn everything you can both in and outside the gym as well. Talk to people who work out regularly. Read various articles and think about what can work for you and what might not. The more prepared you are for your body transformation, the faster you will approach your desired body. If you know exactly what you're doing, your body transformation will be easy for you. Start working hard on yourself and give every repetition 100 percent. Give it your everything and try to improve. One additional rep, five additional pounds or one additional mile. Strive for improvement. Watch your diet and discover what your body likes the most. Discover which meal is best for you before your workout and how much time you need for its digestion and learn how to behave towards your body exactly according to its demands.

## START NOW

Start today. Decide to invest your time into your body transformation now and don't postpone it. People that are hungry for results never procrastinate. If you want to start with your body transformation, start it now. Start going to the gym because that's exactly where you'll be working on your body. Get familiar with the free weights, machines and environment. Start learning the proper exercise form and don't stop for anything. Start now and stay hungry. You've almost read the entire book now. That means you've invested time into your body transformation already. You've started building the base and every new piece of information brings you closer to your ultimate goal. What next steps will you take after you finish reading this book? Will you join a gym? Will you contact a personal trainer? Will you adjust your diet? Decide your next steps now.

## IT'S NEVER TOO LATE

Nothing stands in your way. Not even your age. You can do something at almost every age. Although it's true that, if you're in your fifties, you won't get the efficiency of someone in their twenties, it doesn't mean you shouldn't be active. Just think about how many elderly people run marathons all over the world. They keep their body healthy, strong and functional. It's at this age that you must make sure that your body will continue to serve you well. The principles that your body works upon never change so don't tell yourself: "I'm too old for playing around in the gym. It's too late." Don't write yourself off. You can start any time. It doesn't matter if you're 20 or 50, if you're a student or if you're close to retirement. The possibility of changing your body is always there.

## ENJOY THE PROCESS OF A CHANGE

So start today and enjoy your new adventure. Enjoy every little milestone you achieve and be happy about your progress. Your body transformation is a matter of many little steps; a matter of achieving many smaller milestones that keep you moving forward. One or two additional reps are a success. Lifting heavier than last time is a success. Additional half a mile is a success. Every time you reach new limits, feel happy and be proud of yourself. Don't wait to celebrate until you reach your ultimate goal because this can be a rather long period of time. A month without a great feeling from a job well done is a month too long. Has it been three months? Then it's definitely time to take stock and appreciate what you've done so far. Celebrate every little step forward but take care to keep your discipline high and your ultimate goal on your mind. Celebrate your partial successes but keep moving towards your ultimate goal. If you manage to connect these two things, your body transformation will become an activity that will bring you all kinds of happy moments and will fulfil you as well.

## SUCCESS WITHOUT FULFILMENT IS FAILURE

If you're going to go to a gym, it's important that you feel great about it. There's no doubt that you can transform your body and get exceptional results. The question is whether you'll enjoy it and how much it will fulfil you in the long run. How will you feel after your first month? How will you feel after two months? Will your body transformation fulfil you? If you get results but it doesn't fulfil you, stop. Get some rest and think about why it isn't pleasurable for you. Think about what your workout needs to mean to you in order for you to look forward to it. Think about how to enrich your lifestyle so you get your results and enjoy it at the same time. You're only successful when you have both results and fulfilment. You really need to enjoy it and you need to keep moving forward. It's right then that you feel amazing and you feel you're doing something that's truly a valuable and meaningful part of your life.

## OTHER AREAS OF YOUR LIFE

Whilst you're working towards that final goal, don't neglect the other areas of your life as well. You know, relationships, finance, love, career, fun and spirituality. Find a balance between them. If you focus on something too much and start neglecting the other things, it will soon come to the surface and you will start suffering, which is the last thing you would want for yourself! It'll start in one area and spread like wildfire. You'll start experiencing bad moods and these will spill into other areas. Before you can stop it, you'll find your suffering has cost you too much. So don't focus on only one area of life. Strive for inner balance instead. You will feel good about yourself. You will do your daily activities effortlessly and you will increase the quality of your life. Moreover, your overall satisfaction with your life will reflect onto the success of your body transformation. There is a very close connection between these things.

## A CLOSING WISH

Your journey has begun. I wish you lots of fun and success and I hope your body transformation fulfils you as well. I look forward to when you enjoy that moment after a couple of weeks of hard work, when you look into the mirror and feel happy with your body, knowing the whole process was worth it. If you have before and after photos of your body, email me so I can celebrate with you. After that, get some rest and decide on what to do next. Keep living the healthy lifestyle and keep working out. A strong, healthy and attractive body is one of those things that simply can't be bought.

# Part 6
# Appendices


1. SAMPLE WORKOUT PROGRAMME FOR MUSCLE GAIN

2. SAMPLE WORKOUT PROGRAMME FOR FAT LOSS

3. MUSCLE GAIN DIET SAMPLE; FAT LOSS DIET SAMPLE; SUPPLEMENT PLAN EXAMPLE FOR BOTH MUSCLE GAIN AND FAT LOSS

4. THE SCHOFIELD CALCULATION

# Sample Workout Programme For Muscle Gain

Day 1 - Chest + Triceps

Day 2 - Back + Biceps

Day 3 - Shoulders + Legs

Day 4 - OFF

Day 5 - Chest + Triceps

Day 6 - Back + Biceps

Day 7 - Shoulders + Legs

Day 8 - OFF

Day 9 - OFF

**Day 1 & Day 5 - Chest + Triceps**

Exercise 1 - Benchpress 3x(6-12)

Exercise 2 - Incline Dumbell Press 3x(6-12)

Exercise 3 - Dips 3x(6-12)

Exercise 4 - Tricep Pushdowns 4x(6-12)

Exercise 5 - Skullcrushers 4x(6-12)

**Day 2 & Day 6 - Back + Biceps**

Exercise 1 - Pull Ups 3x(6-12)

Exercise 2 - Bent Over Rows 3x(6-12)

Exercise 3 - Machine Low Row 3x(6-12)

Exercise 4 - Barbel Curls 4x(6-12)

Exercise 5 - Preacher Curls 4x(6-12)

**Day 3 & Day 7 - Shoulders + Legs**

Exercise 1 - Military Press 3x(6-12)

Exercise 2 - Lateral Raises 3x(6-12)

Exercise 3 - Seated Dumbell Press 3x(6-12)

Exercise 4 - Squats 4x(10-15)
Exercise 5 - Leg Press 4x(10-15)
Exercise 6 - Calf Raises 3x(10-15)

**Abs -** Pick two days (e.g. Chest + Biceps = Day 1 & Day 5) and perform your ab exercises at the end of your workout. Use following exercises:

Exercise 1 – Swiss ball Crunches 3x(15-20)
Exercise 2 - Rope Crunches 3x(15-20)
Exercise 3 - Reversed Crunches 3x(15-20)

**Notes -** Rest Interval between individual sets and exercises = 30-90 sec
Total workout time on a training day = 45 minutes excluding warm up, cool down & stretching

Don't forget to warm up before your workout and have a cool down with stretching after your workout.

To avoid a plateau, you might need to change a couple of exercises after 6-8 weeks.

# Sample Workout Programme For Fat Loss

Day 1 - Fullbody A
Day 2 - Cardio
Day 3 - Fullbody B
Day 4 - Cardio
Day 5 - Fullbody C
Day 6 - Cardio
Day 7 – OFF

### Day 1 - Fullbody A

Exercise 1 - Benchpress 3x6-12
Exercise 2 - Pullups 3x6-12
Exercise 3 - Military Press 3x6-12
Exercise 4 - Squats 3x10-15
Exercise 5 - Barbell Curls 3x6-12
Exercise 6 - Rope Crunches 3x15-20
Followed by 10-15 minutes of cardio

### Day 3 - Fullbody B

Exercise 1 - Deadlifts 3x10-15
Exercise 2 - Dumbbell Incline Bench Press 3x6-12
Exercise 3 - Bent Over Rows 3x6-12
Exercise 4 - Lateral Raises 3x6-12
Exercise 5 - Tricep Pushdowns 3x6-12
Exercise 6 – Crunches 3x15-20
Followed by 10-15 minutes of cardio

### Day 4 – Fullbody C

Exercise 1 - Chin-ups 3x6-12
Exercise 2 - Dips 3x6-12
Exercise 3 - Lunges 3x10-15
Exercise 4 - Front Raises 3x6-12

Exercise 5 - Calf Raises 3x15-20
Exercise 6 - Wood Chops 3x10 each side
Followed by 10-15 minutes of cardio

**Cardio** – Your non-workout cardio should be longer than 30 minutes but shorter than 60 minutes - ideally to 45 minutes. Keep the intensity low and your heart rate between 120-140 bps.

**Notes** - Rest Interval between individual sets and exercises = 60-120 sec
    Total workout time on a training day = 60 minutes excluding warm up, cool down & stretching

Don't forget to include warm up, cool down & stretching into your workout.

Tweak your programme after 6-8 weeks to prevent a plateau.

<u>**Muscle Gain Diet Sample for a 70-kg, moderately-active male aged 18-29**</u>

First of all, we need to determine the daily energy expenditure. To do this, we will use the Schofield Calculation.

BMR (Basal Metabolic Rate) = 15.1x70+692 = 1749; PAF (Physical Activity Factor) = 1.7; BMR x PAF = 3000 kcal

For muscle gain, we need to create a caloric surplus so we will add another 300 kcal a day to begin with. The total caloric intake will therefore be around 3300 kcal a day for this person.

**Calorie source and macro-nutrient guidelines:**

Total Protein Intake (2g per 1kg of bodyweight) = 140g of protein = 560 kcal
Total Carbohydrate Intake (7.5g per 1kg of bodyweight) = 530g of carbohydrates = 2110 kcal
Total Fat Intake (1g per 1kg of bodyweight) = 70g of fat = 630 kcal

<u>**Fat Loss Diet Sample for a 80-kg, sedentary female aged 18-29**</u>

Again, we need to determine the daily energy expenditure and will use the Schofield Calculation.

BMR = 14.8x80+487 = 1671; PAF (Physical Activity Factor) = 1.4; BMR x PAF = 2340 kcal

For fat loss, we need to create a caloric deficit so we will take out 300 kcal a day for start. The total caloric intake will therefore be around 2040 kcal a day for this person.

**Calorie source and macro-nutrient guidelines:**

Total Protein Intake (2g per 1kg of bodyweight) = 160g of protein = 640 kcal

Total Carbohydrate Intake (2.1g per 1kg of bodyweight) = 170g of carbohydrates = 680 kcal

Total Fat Intake (1g per 1kg of bodyweight) = 80g of fat = 720 kcal

**<u>Supplement Plan Example for both muscle gain and fat loss</u>**

| Supplements used | Time | Amount |
|---|---|---|
| Whey Protein | 30 minutes before workout, immediately after workout | 1 scoop (25 grams) |
| Creatine Monohydrate | immediately after workout | 5 grams |
| Glucose | immediately after workout | ¾ scoop (15 grams) |
| Multivitamin (capsules) | Morning | As recommended on a label |
| Fish Oil (capsules) | Morning | As recommended on a label |

**The Schofield Calculation**

Men:

| 10 – 17 years | BMR = 17.7 x W + 657 | SEE = 105 |
|---|---|---|
| 18 – 29 years | BMR = 15.1 x W + 692 | SEE = 156 |
| 30 – 59 years | BMR = 11.5 x W + 873 | SEE = 167 |

Women:

| 10 – 17 years | BMR = 13.4 x W + 692 | SEE = 112 |
|---|---|---|
| 18 – 29 years | BMR = 14.8 x W + 487 | SEE = 120 |
| 30 – 59 years | BMR = 8.3 x W + 846 | SEE = 112 |

Key:
W = Body weight in kilograms
SEE = Standard error of estimation


**Physical Activity Factor (PAF)**

BMR x 1.4 – Inactive men and women (sedentary people)
BMR x 1.6  - Moderately active women
BMR x 1.7 – Moderately active men
BMR x 1.8 – Very active women (professional athletes)
BMR x 1.9 – Very active men (professional athletes)

**Example Calculation:**
Let's take the example of a moderately active man aged 18-29 who weighs 70 kg:

BMR = 15.1x70+692 = 1749;

PAF (Physical Activity Factor) = 1.7;

BMR x PAF = **2973 kcal** ± 156 kcal (SEE)

In order to calculate a person's BMR, you need to know their gender, age and weight. First of all, choose one of the two tables according to person's gender and then use the row that relates to their age. Insert their weight into the calculation and you will get their BMR.

The next step is to determine their PAF and multiply their BMR by relevant PAF number. This determines the person's energy expenditure, based on their daily needs and various activities. Please note that there is a standard error of estimation (SEE) that needs to be taken into consideration.  This means that your final calorific result will be within a range.

Taking our example above, our man's final calculation is **2973 kcal** ±156 kcal (SEE). ± means 'plus or minus'.  As such, his actual calorific needs will fall somewhere between 2817 kcal to 3129kcal and it will be up to him to determine what is best for him.

We prepared a special report called
**The Insider's Guide To Super Effective Fat Loss**
Get it on our website www.juggro.com for **FREE**.

Thank you for reading this book.
If you want to take your body transformation even further,
check our amazing Juggro PT board game.

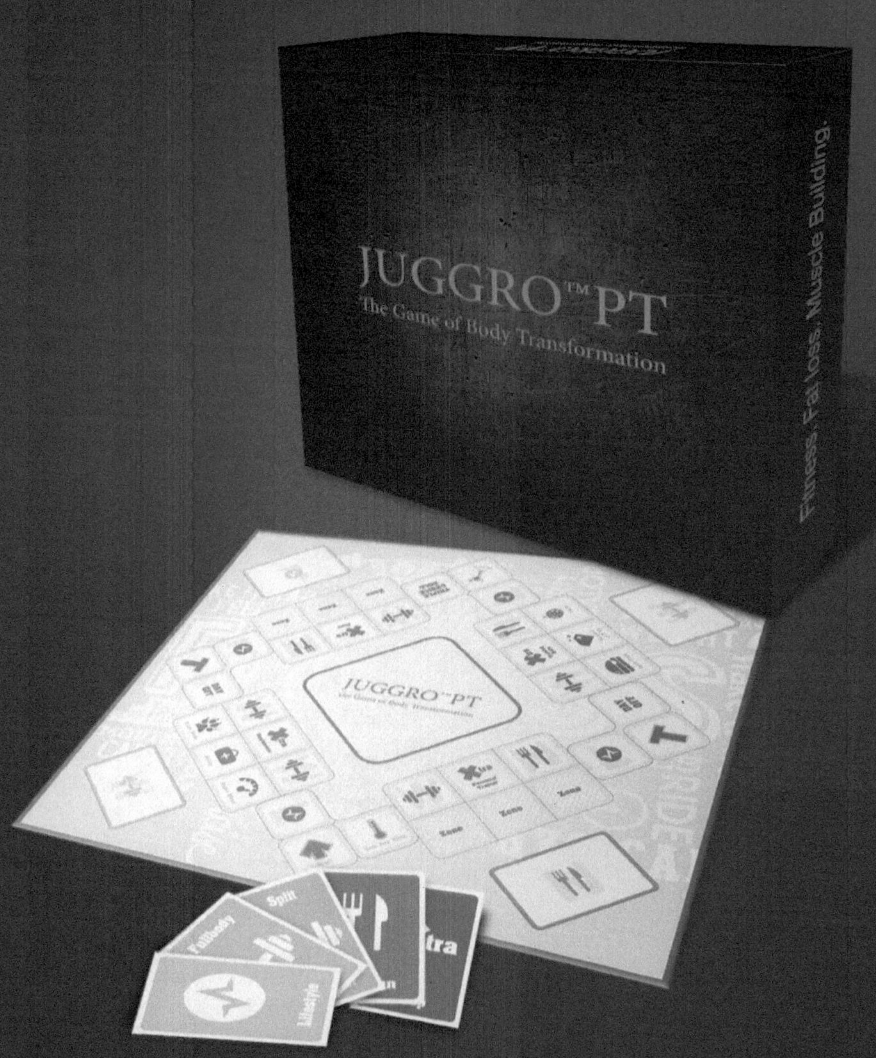


**FIRST TO GAIN OR LOSE**
**20 POUNDS WINS!**

www.ingramcontent.com/pod-product-compliance
Lightning Source LLC
LaVergne TN
LVHW091506170726
843492LV00001B/371